Care Work

Present and Future

Edited by
Janet Boddy, Claire Cameron and
Peter Moss

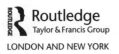

Routledge
Taylor & Francis Group

LONDON AND NEW YORK

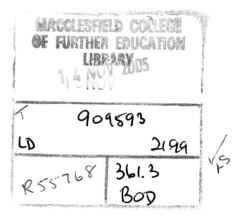
First published 2006
by Routledge
2 Park Square, Milton Park, Abingdon, Oxon OX14 4RN

Simultaneously published in the USA and Canada
by Routledge
270 Madison Ave, New York, NY 10016

Routledge is an imprint of the Taylor & Francis Group

© 2006 Janet Boddy, Claire Cameron and Peter Moss

Typeset in Sabon by RefineCatch Ltd, Bungay, Suffolk
Printed and bound in Great Britain by
Cromwell Press, Trowbridge, Wiltshire

British Library Cataloguing in Publication Data
A catalogue record for this book is available
from the British Library

Library of Congress Cataloging in Publication Data
Boddy, Janet, 1969–
  Care work : present & future / Janet Boddy, Claire Cameron & Peter Moss.
    p. cm.
  Includes bibliographical references
1. Human services – Great Britain.   2. Caregivers – Great Britain.   3.
Social workers – Great Britain.   I. Cameron, Claire.   II. Moss, Peter,
1945–   III. Title.
  HV245.B65 2005
  361.3′0941 – dc22   2005008210

ISBN 0–415–34772–6 (hbk)
ISBN 0–415–34773–4 (pbk)

Contents

vi *Contents*

Illustrations

Acknowledgements

The views expressed in this book belong to its authors, but the research on which it is based was made possible by the support of a variety of funders, to whom we express our thanks: the European Union; the Joseph Rowntree Foundation; the Economic and Social Research Council; the Nuffield Foundation; and several English government departments: the Department of Health; the Home Office; the Department for Education and Skills; and the Youth Justice Board.

The editors are grateful to colleagues at Thomas Coram Research Unit for their support in the development and writing of this book, to Michelle Cage for her patience and tenacity in compiling the bibliography, among other editorial assistance, and in particular to Peter Aggleton for his timely and ever-insightful feedback.

Preface

In late 2002, the authors of this book gathered, as a group of colleagues at Thomas Coram Research Unit (TCRU), to discuss their work. TCRU is a multidisciplinary research unit within the Institute of Education, University of London, founded by Jack Tizard in 1973. Over recent years, the Unit has undertaken a wide range of research into care work and care workers, but we (the authors) felt that there had been too little discussion across projects, and so there was a risk that our knowledge could be to some extent fragmented, no more than the sum of its parts. We wanted to bring this work together, and to a wider audience, and in doing so, to build on *Rethinking Children's Care* (Brannen and Moss 2003), an earlier volume that collected different strands of work at TCRU. The result is before you, *Care Work: Present and Future*.

Our aim in producing this book was not to update *Rethinking Children's Care*, nor simply to collect accounts of a variety of research studies that happen to have been conducted at TCRU. This volume addresses the whole life course (although, as befits the Unit's remit, much of our work has been focused on children and young people), and stands alongside another Routledge volume, *In Care and After: A Positive Perspective* (Chase et al. forthcoming), which is based on research conducted at TCRU with young people who are looked after. Furthermore, while the *Care Work* book draws on particular pieces of work, it is built around specific key questions highlighted in chapter 1, and explored in the first part of the book, and subsequently discussed in relation to the specific examples of care work that form Part II. This goal necessitated a different, less individualised, approach to writing than is usually the case with edited volumes. That meeting in 2002 proved to be the first of many (bolstered by biscuits and cups of tea), as part of a collaborative and discursive process during which ideas, and progressive drafts of chapters, were discussed and refined by all the book's authors. For us, as editors, this process has been as rewarding as it has been effective, in creating a volume characterised by cross-referencing of common themes, shared understandings and collectively arrived at conclusions.

Janet Boddy, Claire Cameron and Peter Moss

Part I

1 Care work, present and future

Introduction

*Peter Moss, Janet Boddy and
Claire Cameron*

Care work – the concept in question

This book is about work referred to today in the United Kingdom (UK),[1] both in policy and everyday language, as 'care' – childcare (both in centres and family day care), home or domiciliary care, residential care, foster care and (sometimes used as a blanket term) social care. It is about the people who are engaged in this work, both paid workers, whether employees or self-employed, and unpaid workers, including relatives, friends and neighbours and volunteers. It is about who these workers are; what their work entails, including both activities and relationships; their conditions of work and where they work; and the education and knowledge they require and receive. Focused mainly on the UK, the book draws on experience from other countries, to demonstrate how care work can be differently conceptualised and structured and, in so doing, to raise questions about taken-for-granted assumptions.

This confident statement of intent, however, masks an uncertainty and ambivalence that runs through the book. 'Care work' is a widely recognised term, and 'care workers', paid and unpaid, are a numerous group undertaking socially important tasks. Despite working in different settings and with different groups, we shall argue that care workers have a number of important features in common. Yet at the same time, the validity and usefulness of the concept of 'care work' is in question throughout the book. Indeed, in our concluding chapter we address the question of whether care work has a future, by which we mean should it continue to be treated as a separate field for policy and employment purposes?

There are several reasons for calling the concept into question. The first is that areas referred to as care work in the UK are not always regarded as such in other countries, but may be located elsewhere within different policy and employment fields. This comes about in various ways. The borders between care and other fields are becoming increasingly blurred. In the case of work with elderly people, it is the borders between care, housing and health. While in the case of work with children, it is the border between care and education that is increasingly indistinct, sometimes to the point of disappearing altogether. An example concerns 'childcare' services for preschool children, which in countries such as New Zealand and Sweden are now treated as an integral part of the education system. In these cases, 'childcare' and education are treated as inseparable, while 'childcare workers' are replaced by a new type of teacher, educated to work with children from birth up to school age, working alongside another group of workers with a lower level of education. In Sweden these 'early years' teachers currently make up about half the early years workforce, while the goal in New Zealand is for all the staff in most types of early years services to be teachers by 2012 (Cohen et al. 2004; New Zealand Ministry of Education 2002).

Alternatively, care work may never have been a separate field of policy and employment, or at least not for many years. A prime example, which forms the subject of chapter 6, is the profession of *pedagogue* (or *educateur* in French), widespread in continental Europe and found working in a range of occupations that in Britain would be considered 'care work'. The most wide-ranging example is the Danish pedagogue, the mainstay of the workforce in what we in Britain would term 'childcare' services – preschool and school-age – and in a wide range of occupations in what we would term 'social care', from residential services for children and young people, through services for younger adults with severe disabilities to, though less common, work with elderly people. The Danish pedagogue can truly lay claim to being able to work with people from birth to 100 and increasingly beyond 100! Underlying this profession is a theory and practice of pedagogy grounded in a holistic approach to the child and adult and to the provision of services in which care cannot be separated from a broad concern with well-being and (in the case of children and young people) upbringing.

These examples involve 'care work' as a separate entity in policy, with care services being reconceptualised out of existence, or never being present in the first place. But the concept of care work is being squeezed in other ways. Take, for example, the case of direct payment schemes, where the 'cared for' person receives cash benefits with which to pay for workers they select, organise and employ rather than services organised and delivered by public agencies. These schemes are now spreading across many countries and across areas previously defined as social care for adults, starting with younger adults with disabilities and extending to elderly people. This policy change has been, in part, the product of a rights movement that has called for the empowerment of people with disabilities by giving them direct control over the resources needed to live an independent life. In the process, they have rejected the concept and language of care as implying dependency and dropped the term 'care worker' or 'home carer' in favour of 'personal assistant'.

The second reason for questioning 'care work' is that the term 'care' is often weakly conceptualised in policy and practice, so that its meaning is unclear. For instance, the term 'social care' is frequently used in the UK to define policy and employment and to name key policy-related bodies: e.g. the Commission for Social Care Inspection, the Social Care Institute for Excellence, the Social Care Workforce Research Unit and the General Social Care Council (all from England), or the UK Sector Skills Council for Social Care, Children and Young People. Yet it is rare to find any definition or discussion of its meaning in policy documents or on organisations' websites.

Even when the English minister responsible for adult social care announced in 2004 that he 'wanted to develop a new vision for social care', no attention was paid then or in the subsequent consultation to defining the term – 'social care' was simply taken for granted (Social Care Institute of Excellence 2004). Moreover, as we shall see in chapter 4, workers in the 'social care' sector find it difficult if not impossible to define what the term means. Not surprisingly, therefore, a recent think tank report on the 'social care workforce' admits that 'defining exactly what social care *is* continues to vex practitioners and policymakers alike . . . [and is] a term that generates neither recognition among the general public, nor affection among staff' (Roche and Rankin 2004: 5 original emphasis). The authors are thrown back on the argument that, in practice, social care is defined by shared values. However, it is unclear how exactly the values specified – 'achieving social inclusion and better life opportunities for vulnerable people' (Roche and Rankin 2004) – are specific to a group labelled 'social care workers'. Might not many other groups say that such values were important to them too?

In practice, at a policy and service level, 'social care' is used as a descriptive label, serving as an umbrella term for labelling a wide range of services. For example, on the website for the Department of Health (https//www.dh.gov.uk), the English ministry which deals with adult social care, the page headed 'about social care' offers this short statement by way of explanation:

> The term 'social care' covers a wide range of services, which are provided by local authorities and the independent sector. Social care comes in many forms, such as care at home, in day centres or by way of residential or nursing homes. The term also covers services such as providing meals on wheels to the elderly, home help for people with disabilities and fostering services.

The meaning of the term 'social care' has received more attention academically. In its broadest usage, 'social care' is a concept that covers the life course and spans many boundaries (Ungerson 1997): formal and informal care, paid and unpaid, public and private – and children and adults. A recent European research project specifically on social care defines the concept in this broad transcendent sense as:

> assistance that is provided in order to help children or adult people with the activities of their daily lives and it can be provided either as paid or as unpaid work, by professionals or non-professionals and it can

take place as well in the public as in the private sphere. In particular, it is distinctive to social care that it transcends the conceptual dichotomies between the public and the private, the professional and the non-professional, the paid and the unpaid.

(Kroger 2001: 4)

This concept of 'social care' has been most often used in research, especially feminist analysis of welfare regimes. It provides, it has been argued, a basis for developing comparative analyses of such regimes with a strong gender perspective (Daly and Lewis 1999). From this perspective, an important issue is where the line is actually drawn in welfare states – between private and public responsibility for social care, between unpaid and paid work – and the implications for the gendering of care work.

We see care as an activity with costs, both financial and emotional, which extend across public/private boundaries. The important analytic questions that arise in this regard centre upon how the costs involved are shared, among individuals, families and within society at large. Our three-dimensional approach leads us to define social care as the activities and relations involved in meeting the physical and emotional requirements of dependent adults and children, and the normative, economic and social frameworks within which these are assigned and carried out.

(Daly and Lewis 1999: 285)

Conceptualised in this way, 'social care' can be seen as an activity that has been mainly undertaken by women in the home, disadvantaging them in the labour market. To free women to participate in the labour market on equal terms with men, policies are needed which move this activity of 'social care' – and therefore its costs – into the public domain. From a gender perspective, the issue is how far welfare states enable 'defamilialisation', that is policies, and in particular the provision of care services, 'that lessen individuals' reliance on family; that maximise individuals' command of economic resources independently of familial or conjugal reciprocities' (Esping-Andersen 1999: 45).

Understood in this way, 'social care' is a similar activity wherever it takes place or whoever undertakes the activity and whether or not the work is paid: the paid care worker and the unpaid (female) carer are interchangeable. 'Care work', when defined as paid care, is viewed as the commodification of the work of housewives, mothers, and other family members; their unpaid work is done instead by paid workers. This concept of 'care work' has much in common with another concept – 'household services' – which includes care (childcare and eldercare) alongside other household tasks such as cooking and cleaning (Yeandle et al. 1999). These tasks are bracketed together as work that has been primarily undertaken within households by female members, on an unpaid basis, but are all potentially capable of substitution by paid workers, when the performance of these tasks becomes 'household services'. The interest here of the European Union, and others is in 'household services' as a source of increased employment.

This transcendent concept of 'social care' (or 'household services'), therefore, embodies a very particular and contentious assumption. Formal care services and paid care workers are implicitly understood as replicating the home and informal household carers, such as mothers. Nurseries and other services for young children, for example, may seek to be – or be seen to be – substitute homes, and carers in these services substitute mothers (Dahlberg et al. 1999). Paid care of elderly people, it has been argued, may best be undertaken by women drawing on their domestic skills and experience acquired as housewives (Wærness 1982, 1995).

This way of conceptualising social care has its value. It draws our attention to the important matter of how work with children and adults, and the associated costs, is allocated between family, market and state and between women and men. But whether used in descriptive or transcendent mode, 'social care' has little to contribute to an understanding of 'care work' itself, what different groups of care worker do or might do, whether and how unpaid care work may differ from paid care work, and whether 'care work' is a useful term for purposes of policy, provision and practice.

We could make a similar case for the weak concept of care in other areas, such as 'childcare'. The point at issue is that weak conceptualisation – not being able to give a well-argued explanation of what 'care' means, including what qualities and features make it distinctive – leaves 'care work' very open to being redefined and repositioned. A weak concept, therefore, makes a poor foundation on which to build policy and advance practice.

It could also be added that it is difficult to draw clear boundaries for a weak or indistinct concept. For example, should we include jobs designated as 'customer care'? Should classroom assistants, a rapidly growing occupational group, be considered care workers, even though 'care' is not in their job title and they work in the field of education? Does nursing today merit inclusion as 'care work' and if so does this apply equally to fully qualified nurses and the various groups of nursing assistant? In practice we have excluded all of these groups, but these exclusions are contestable.

A third reason for questioning the concept is that, to maintain the analogy, it seems to support a rather poor and flimsy building: as we shall see, for example in chapters 2 and 5, employment conceptualised and described as 'care work' is usually associated with low levels of qualification, low pay and low status. Removed from the care work field and placed in another, such as education or pedagogy, employment is much more valued. To take an extreme instance, Danish pedagogues working in nurseries are graduates and earn more than twice as much as their British 'childcare' counterparts who are unlikely to have been educated beyond an upper secondary level.

Of course, this is more than a simple matter of renaming: deciding to call

UK childcare workers pedagogues would not change their position. But it points to the implications of a job being understood in terms of 'care'; if that job were to be reconceptualised, to be understood for example in terms of education or health, then it is likely to be revalued. Here, the significance of understanding 'social care' as replication of care performed at home becomes clear. While employment is understood as 'simply' substituting for unpaid work done by women in the home, it is likely to suffer the social devaluation attached to unpaid home work and to be viewed as do-able by any woman because of innate 'caring' qualities and prior domestic experience.

Having voiced our doubts at this early stage about the concept of 'care work', we should be equally clear that we are not rejecting the importance of 'care' in work with people. Indeed we would argue that 'care' is too marginalised at present and should figure prominently in many work areas where currently it has little or no recognition. Our argument, which we will develop in concluding this volume, is that perhaps the care in work with people should be seen and practised as an ethic – an ethic of care, which in the words of Tronto (1993) 'involves particular acts of caring and a "general habit of mind" to care that should inform all aspects of moral life' (Tronto 1993: 127), both caring for and caring about.

Taking a life course, historical and cross-national perspective

This book is wide-ranging in its scope. We do not claim to deal with every facet of 'care work', nor to pay equal attention to all those facets that we do include: overall, we devote more space to work with children and young people than to work with adults. But we do cover areas of 'care work' that span the life course, from care work with young children to care work with very elderly people. In our approach and thinking, we attempt to keep the life course in view and to look for connections between care work with people at different stages of the life course.

We also span different forms of care work: paid workers in services (varying themselves from professional workers such as the pedagogues featured in chapter 6 to lowly qualified workers such as family day carers, who use their own home as a site for childcare work, discussed in chapter 5); volunteers working for no money (such as many of the mentors featured in chapter 7) and private foster carers whose income from their work often covers little more than their expenses, if that (featured in chapter 8); and unpaid workers caring for family members (the subject of chapter 9). But these are not mutually exclusive categories. Thus, women may enter paid care work as a direct result of becoming or being informal carers: family day carers, for example, typically enter the work when they have their own young children since they want employment that will enable them to be at home and care for their own children (Mooney et al. 2001). Or, to take another example, women often enter social care (such as work with elderly people) because the hours enable them to combine this employment with their personal care responsibilities, be it for children or elderly relatives (Johansson and Moss 2004).

Nor are these categories, and the work that falls into each, fixed. There is much fluidity in care work, with changes taking place over time. It is important, therefore, to recognise the temporal specificity of any analysis of care work and the need for a historical perspective. While our historical perspective in most parts of the book is relatively short term, covering at most a few decades, chapter 3 takes a longer term view, exploring nineteenth-century understandings of care using novels to demonstrate how 'care and care work are the products of specific social contexts . . . and relate to governing ideologies'. Not only do the amount and type of care work change over time, with changes for example in employment, health and population structure; but so, too, does the availability of care workers (a point to which we shall return shortly) and views about who these care workers should be (changing views about men and care feature strongly in chapter 3) and what qualities and qualifications they need for the work.

Sometimes, certain types of work move out of the care field altogether: as already noted, 'childcare' can become 'education'. New forms of work may enter, and existing ones change. Chapter 7 provides one example – mentoring children and young people – where an area of work starts out life undertaken by volunteers, but one possible direction over time may be a shift towards greater formality and professionalisation. Another example of the fluidity of care work, also already noted, is the way 'home care' for adults with disabilities is being recast as 'personal assistance' as a consequence of direct payment schemes; while in some countries, these schemes may be used to employ relatives, creating a hybrid situation where kin, normally unpaid carers, become paid workers. A third example concerns childcare: as chapter 9 describes, grandparents (and mainly grandmothers) are still the main providers of regular childcare in Britain. But this is no longer the case in Denmark and Sweden. This may be due in part to increased employment among women in their 50s; but another reason is the growth of affordable and available formal services, so that in effect paid care work has replaced one type of unpaid care work.

We should, however, be wary of over-simplifying changes underway in the relationship between more formal and more informal care work. While there may be a widespread secular trend from informal to formal care for children, the situation in adult care is less clear-cut; in some countries at least, such as Sweden and the UK, there is a trend to target public care services on fewer, more dependent elderly people, leaving relatives overall to do more caring (Johansson and Moss 2004). Moreover, increasing formal services may reconstitute rather than reduce informal care. In Denmark, for example, grandparents may play little part today in regular childcare arrangements, but they play an important role in providing emergency care (Moss and Cameron 2002). In Norway, another country with a highly developed welfare state, high levels of formal services for elderly people may contribute to new forms of involvement by families, including service promotion, mediation and support (Lingsom 1997).

We should, too, be wary of the distinction we have introduced between 'formal' care work (paid employment conducted in services) and 'informal' care work (unpaid work conducted by family members and friends). In chapter 2, we use this as the starting point for analysing the composition of the care workforce. Yet this dichotomous classification, which mirrors the traditional distinction in social theory between public paid employment and private unpaid labour, is misleading in its simplicity, for example in excluding the 'third sector' voluntary workforce (Taylor 2004). The next chapter, therefore, goes on to explore the variety of 'other' forms of care work that exist in Britain today, largely unpaid but not carried out by family members or friends.

While this 'trichotomous' conceptualisation of care work provides a useful basis for analysing workforce characteristics, it cannot capture fully the complexity of care work. Care work and workers can be differentiated according to the positions they occupy on a number of dimensions, what Lyon (2004) refers to as 'socio-economic modes', such as: the relationship between the care worker and the person cared for; the employment status of the care worker (including, but not only, whether or not they are paid); the extent to which the work is regulated by government agencies or other agencies such as professional bodies; and the level and type of education and qualification needed to practise the work. These modes, in turn, connect with each other in different configurations for different forms of work and different groups of workers. Taking account of these dimensions and connections, it may be more useful to think of different types of care work strung out along a continuum, ranging from very formal (no kin or friendship relationship; the worker as employee or self-employed; the work undertaken within a regulatory framework; the worker educated at tertiary level) to very informal (close kin relationship; the worker not employed; the work outside any regulatory framework; and no entry qualification or training required to undertake the work). Over time, as change occurs in one or more of these dimensions, positioning on the continuum may change. Thus rather than 'formal' care workers, constituting one large block differentiated from another large block of 'informal care workers', we can think of different groups of paid workers positioned at different points towards the more formal end of the continuum depending on education, qualification and extent of regulation; with different groups of unpaid workers spread out along the informal end of the continuum.

As well as a life course and historical perspective, the book also has a cross-national element. While not applied consistently across all chapters, this element is sufficiently present to emphasise how understandings, structures and practices are all produced not only within temporal contexts but also within specific spatial contexts, in societies shaped by particular economic, political, social and cultural forces. Thus, to return to an earlier example, the fact that much of the poorly qualified and paid care work in Britain is well-qualified and quite well-paid pedagogical work in Denmark is not some accident of history. The reasons need to be sought in different traditions (for example, Denmark's close relationship with the continental theory and practice of pedagogy) and in different welfare regimes or relationships between state, market and family – a 'liberal' welfare regime in Britain, a 'Nordic' or 'social democratic' regime in Denmark (Esping-Andersen 1999) – themselves the product of different social and political values.

Such cross-national comparisons both reveal and challenge assumptions in one's own country. They make the familiar strange. They also indicate there are choices to be made when it comes to understandings, structures and practices. At the same time, they throw light on why things are as they are and some of the barriers to change – whilst, hopefully, avoiding the dead end of welfare regime determinism.

A cross-national element in care work is not, however, confined to comparisons of how care work is organised and practised in different countries. Care work itself can cross national borders. Relatives may care for family members normally living far away, for example grandparents in Bangladesh or China can provide substantial though occasional support for adult children and grandchildren living in England (Li 2005). While women from poorer countries provide paid domestic service, often including care work, for families in richer countries (so far migrant labour in formal services, in the UK at least, has been mainly confined to more professionalised fields experiencing labour shortages, such as health services, social work and teaching). Andersen (2000) has described how cross-national care work functions in major European cities, while Hochschild (2000:131), from an American perspective, has written vividly about what she terms 'global care chains'. These are a series of personal links across the globe based on the paid or unpaid work of caring:

> usually women make up these chains . . . [which] usually start in a poor country and end in a rich one . . . [Chains] vary in the number of links – some have one, others two or three – and each link varies in its connective strength. One common form of such a chain is: (1) an older daughter from a poor family who cares for her siblings while (2) her mother works as a nanny caring for the children of a migrating nanny who, in turn (3) cares for the child of a family in a rich country . . . Each kind of chain expresses an invisible human ecology of care, one kind of care depending on another and so on.
>
> (p. 131)

Similarities and convergences

The broad life course approach we adopt in this book has been enabled by the wide range of research and studies undertaken in recent years at the Thomas Coram Research Unit from which the authors of this book have been able to choose. But we have also chosen to take this approach because we believe, on the basis of this wide-ranging research, that certain similarities and connections become apparent when adopting a life course approach that spans care work from birth to 100. We start this section, therefore, by considering some of these similarities and connections, and in the concluding chapter return to the issue when we ask how useful a cross-sectoral approach can be – in policy, training and research.

At the same time, we also know that this can be difficult terrain. There is much territoriality, so trespassers risk prosecution. Insularity often breeds misunderstandings and misconceptions (as with the accusation that by looking at both services for young children and elderly people, you may contribute to 'infantilising' elderly people). We are also aware of adopting a cross-sectoral approach at a moment, in Britain at least, when the *Zeitgeist* is greater integration: between services for children and between services for adults. This is epitomised by the transfer over the last decade in England and Scotland of non-health children's services from health and welfare departments to education departments. This has included 'childcare' and children's 'social care', leaving health and welfare departments to focus on adult 'social care' services. This process, therefore, has a double dynamic: closer relations between services for particular age groups and, at the same time, a widening divide between services for different age groups, in particular children and young people on the one side and adults on the other.

Yet even as this divide – between care work for children and adults – widens (at least in Britain), there remain important similarities that, in our view, merit more cross-sectoral exchanges and connections. First, care workers themselves have much in common. Most paid care work in Britain today is found in the private sector, following deliberate policies to contract the public sector's role as provider and to encourage the provision of new services as businesses; in 2003, 85 per cent of British nurseries (Laing and Buisson 2004), a majority of residential homes for children and young people and 91 per cent of adult care homes (for elderly people or younger adults) (Laing and Buisson 2004) were run by private and voluntary providers, mostly for profit. National standards covering care services, whether for children or adults, require a low level of workforce qualification; for example, level 2 in childcare and eldercare (equivalent to a secondary level qualification), and even this low level is not a requirement for all workers. Surveys of the workforces in various areas of care work show that levels of actual qualification are also rather low (Simon et al. 2003).

As subsequent chapters show clearly, care work of whatever type is largely women's work, even more so in paid than unpaid work. Indeed, care work is one of the most gendered areas of work in the economy. Paid work with young children and elderly adults has the highest proportion of women workers. Men are most likely to be found working with older children, young people and younger adults or caring for elderly spouses.

Reliance on women workers with low levels of qualification across care work sectors creates a second similarity, a shared dilemma: an increasing demand for paid workers (as more children and elderly people require services) at a time when the main source of labour supply (women with low educational qualifications) is diminishing and alternative employment sources have been opening up for them for example, in retail and other parts of the private non-care service sector. Coomans (2002) has described the likely consequences of the end of an era when the economic system in Europe was based on an abundant labour supply:

> This will change thoroughly the behaviour of the labour market and force us to unheard of organisational innovation . . . The number of young people aged 15–24 (in the EU) will be below the number aged 55–64 by 2007, meaning no possible overall replacement of the older working generations by young incomers – with a similar picture for candidate states. . . .

> [With falling numbers of people with low qualifications] all investments and work organisations based on low skill/low wage strategies will face ever-increasing difficulties in terms of labour supply . . .

> The lesson that should be drawn from this is the following: *wherever the present standard for any category of job is 'low qualified women around the age of 30', there will unmistakably be a strong need to improve the quality of job so it will be acceptable to people with higher educational attainments. And if no improved professionalisation of the job was achieved, then it will rapidly end up in a severe labour supply shortage.*

> (Coomans 2002:1, 2, 5, 6, 8: emphasis added)

Faced by these changes, at the heart of which are profound changes in women's education and employment, 'care work' in the twenty-first century could be heading for a crisis, unless new sources of cheap labour are found and exploited or radical changes are made to the work itself including greatly improved education and pay. We return to consider these options and the wider 'crisis of care' argument in our concluding chapter.

We have already referred to the low level of qualification required across much care work in Britain, whether with children or adults. But another similarity across different types of paid care work relates to the type of training leading to qualification, what is termed in chapter 4, an 'industrial-vocational' model: focused on particular tasks in specific services, with employer-defined 'occupational standards' and workplace-based training intended to enable workers to show competence in meeting these standards. Furthermore, the 'care workforce', whether in services for children or adults, is structured around a multitude of occupations without a professional superstructure bringing some cohesion to these disparate occupations.

These particular features of the care workforce can be brought more sharply into focus by contrasting, again, the situation in Britain and Denmark, a comparison developed further in chapter 4. In Denmark, the workforce across most of what we would term 'care services' is also structured around a variety of occupations; but, unlike Britain, in most occupations most workers are drawn from a single profession, the pedagogue. Moreover the initial education of the pedagogue is academically based, taking place in an institute of higher education, albeit with a strong emphasis on practice. A Danish pedagogue working with young children in a nursery might have spent some time previously working with adults with disabilities and might plan to move on to work in a residential service for young people; in Britain, 'care workers' could not move readily between such different occupations.

One rationale for having a cross-sectoral professional worker in Denmark is that certain common qualities and capabilities are seen as necessary across a wide range of settings and with diverse groups of people: children, young people and adults. This is now coming to be recognised in England, at least with respect to work with children and young people: a recent Green Paper, for example, speaks of enabling 'all people working with children to share a common core of skills, knowledge and competence' (Department for Education and Skills 2003: 92), and work on this common core is proceeding. So far, though, there has been no such recognition of similarities across work with children and adults. However, we believe there are similarities, a subject to which we return in the concluding chapter.

Differences and divergences

If we look at care work, both in Britain and more widely across Europe, striking differences can be discerned within the field covered in this book. In most cases, paid work with children and young people on the one hand and with adults on the other is structurally divided with, as we have seen, the divide growing wider in some cases. There is also a status divide: the status of much paid work with children is higher than that with adults and especially elderly people, reflected most obviously in higher levels of training. Indeed, in some countries (notably the Nordic states) much employment in what in Britain is termed 'childcare work' has been raised to a graduate profession, either as a teacher or pedagogue. Moreover, the gap between adultcare and childcare is probably widening (Moss and Cameron 2002).

What might account for this difference? One explanation is the social value of the 'care receivers'. Wærness (1980) has classified what she defines as care work into three categories. In the first category, she counts care work that can be related to growth or some outcome – a result. Work with children who are going to be grown ups and assume responsibility for themselves, as well as be the future labour force, is one example. In the second category, Wærness counts care for people that aims to maintain the status quo, for example treatment of people with disabilities or chronic illnesses. In the third category, she puts care work that is tied to decline – work without any apparent result. The clearest example of this is the way in which care work with elderly people may often be perceived.

If we follow this schema, then two points are apparent. First, services for the first group, and especially for children, are attracting increasing public funds, both to expand the quantity of provision and to improve its quality. So across Europe, childcare services are expanding, with universal provision for children over three years (in kindergarten or nursery school) either achieved or within sight: the European Union has even established quantitative targets, the so-called Barcelona targets, requiring member states to provide childcare places for 33 per cent of children under three years and 90 per cent of children from three to compulsory school age by 2012. At the same time, investment in staffing is increasing, as more emphasis is placed on the educational and developmental role of services; levels of training for childcare services have risen in recent years in many countries. In contrast to this shift to universal publicly-funded services for children, care of elderly people still relies heavily on the private sphere, mostly family but also elderly people purchasing their own services. As we have already noted, the trend in countries such as England and Sweden has been to concentrate publicly-funded services on elderly people with the highest levels of dependency, in contrast to the universalising trend apparent in services for children.

Care work, or at least informal care work, with children and with elderly, sick or disabled adults has different trajectories. As chapter 9 shows, the former is usually anticipated, continuous, time limited and following a predictable course, marked by the child's growing independence. By contrast, the latter may be unexpected, intermittent and unpredictable in course and duration, but often increasing in intensity as the care recipient becomes more dependent.

A second distinction can be defined within the care work field, related to the location of the work. Much paid care work is undertaken in institutions, which in turn divide between those providing day care and residential care. But a substantial amount is undertaken in domestic housing, either that of the carer (family day carers, foster carers) or that of the person cared for (nannies, home carers, personal assistants). Care work in domestic settings usually has the lowest status, possibly because it is most closely associated with family care and domestic service. It also incurs complex boundary issues arising, for example, when a carer works in another person's house, when a carer admits someone else's children into her own home, when a paid carer is a parent herself, and when trying to combine the roles of care worker and businesswoman. Some of these, and other, border issues are explored in greater detail in chapter 5, which focuses on the location of care work, and in chapter 8, which considers a particular group of domestic care workers about whom little is known: private foster carers.

A third distinction concerns the relationship – assumed and actual – between the cared-for person and the care worker. In unpaid care work, the relationships between, for example, young child and parent and between adult child and elderly parent are very different. In paid care work, too, very different relationships are encountered. In the case of childcare services in a private market system such as in Britain, young children can be seen as placed and paid for by their parents who are assumed to be customers purchasing the commodity of childcare. The same is true for private fostering. But in public fostering and residential care for children and young people, the customer is the public authority seeking a placement for a looked-after charge. While in the case of care work with adults, it is more likely to be the cared-for person who seeks services and is the customer. This is most apparent in direct payment schemes, where people with disabilities receive cash benefits to pay directly for the services they need.

Of course in practice these distinctions are not so clear cut. The increasing importance attached to children's rights and participation has led to more emphasis on the relationship between children and services; in less market-oriented countries, access to services can be viewed as an entitlement of children (Cohen et al. 2004). Furthermore, family members often play a mediating role in the relationship between adults and care services.

The rest of this book

The Thomas Coram Research Unit (TCRU) at the Institute of Education, University of London was founded in 1973. Its first director, Professor Jack Tizard, was one of the UK's leading post-war social researchers. While its initial work, and most of its current work, is concerned with children, young people and families, in recent years research has been undertaken into care work involving adults with disabilities and with elderly people. Another feature of TCRU's work has been a strong cross-national dimension, in particular in other parts of Europe. This has led, for example, to an interest in and study of the theory and practice of pedagogy and the profession of pedagogue.

This book, authored by researchers at TCRU, draws on research undertaken into care work over the last 10 years, and exploits both the cross-sectoral and cross-national dimensions of that work: readers can find short summaries of TCRU research studies referred to in the Appendix. The chapters that follow are organised into two parts. After an overview of the care workforce in chapter 2, chapters 3 to 5 each focus on a particular cross-cutting theme: historical understandings, education and location. The book, in its second part, then changes direction. Chapters 6 to 9 turn from cross-cutting themes to focus on four particular groups of care workers located at different points on what we have referred to as the care work continuum, ranging from informal family carers to the profession of pedagogue, with private foster carers and mentors positioned between these extremes.

The book ends by returning to pick up some of the issues already aired in this chapter. In particular it will consider whether 'care work' has a future as a separate policy and employment field and whether a crisis in care work is in the offing and, if so, how it might be averted. This second issue – the crisis of care question – will require particular attention to the relationship between care work and gender. We conclude by considering what direction paid care work might take over the first part of this century, reflecting on cross-sectoral similarities in paid work and the relative merits of generalist or specialist training. This exercise in futurology is intended to provoke the reader into considering the possibilities in a century when care work will be as important as ever, whilst the foundations on which care work in the twentieth century was based – in particular an endless reserve of unpaid or low paid female labour – have subsided and crumbled.

Note

1 The United Kingdom consists of four nations or parts: England, Northern Ireland, Scotland and Wales. Although they share much in common, there are some differences in policy, provision and practice. Throughout the book we have attempted to make it clear when we refer to the United Kingdom, Great Britain (i.e. the UK less Northern Ireland) or particular nations (e.g. England).

2 Who are today's care workers?

Antonia Simon and Charlie Owen

Introduction

The question of who are today's care workers is complex, involving decisions about how care work is defined, what types of work are done by care workers, for whom the care work is done, how organised the work is, and whether the work is paid or unpaid or somewhere in between the two. Care work can be considered along a continuum: at one end are those people carrying out care work as a formal paid occupation (the formal care workforce). At the other, there are those who do caring work as an activity without pay or formal employment structures (informal care workers). However, there is much fluidity in the construct and practice of care work, and these different categories of care worker are neither fixed nor mutually exclusive. Moreover, along this continuum are those whose care work shares features of formal and informal care. Examples include voluntary workers, including mentors who may be formally organised but unpaid, or paid expenses rather than salaries, and foster carers who are paid expenses but not usually employed. For the purposes of the discussion in this chapter, these varied roles will be considered together as 'other care workers', while acknowledging that their differences are as many as their commonalities.

In this chapter, we explore the characteristics of the care workforce in Great Britain[1] today, primarily with reference to national statistics from regular surveys. This chapter will present a picture of those engaged in formal, informal, and other forms of care work, derived from statistical data about their characteristics and working conditions. In doing so, it will examine the usefulness of these categorisations of care worker, and thus set the scene for subsequent chapters, which will explore, in more depth, understandings of different forms of care work.

To identify care workers using national statistical data is to define them in terms of the work they do, paid or unpaid. Discussion of the formal care workforce is based on occupational categorisations in census and Labour Force Survey data; information about informal care workers is drawn from national surveys such as the General Household Survey and the census, based on information about those who provide 'help or support' to others.

Those that we have categorised as 'other care workers' cannot be identified from national statistics, and so this element of the discussion is based on other quantitative, but non-national, research evidence.

The formal care workforce

The care work being carried out by the formal workforce is done as part of their job. This group is, therefore, relatively easy to identify within published statistics that include occupation, because care workers can be recognised by their occupation. Formal care work is characterised by the exchange of payment for a set of services, by the formal organisation of the work (usually a pre-agreed time, place and duration for the work being carried out) and by a formally defined relationship between the person being cared for and the person being paid to provide the care.

The approach taken in this part of the chapter draws on a major Thomas Coram Research Unit study, entitled *Mapping the Care Workforce* (Simon et al. 2003), which was funded by the Department of Health. The formal care workforce was defined for this work by *occupations* using the Standard Occupational Classifications (SOC) (Office for National Statistics 2000). The SOC is a detailed classification of occupations comprised of hundreds of unit groups. Unit groups are sets of specific occupations, grouped together on the basis of tasks performed, qualifications, training, skills and experience commonly associated with those tasks. Occupations were chosen on the basis of their descriptions as those providing direct, 'hands on' care: managers and others indirectly involved in the workforce were excluded. We only included those occupations providing social care, excluding other forms of care, such as medical care provided by doctors and the care provided by nurses. We have divided these occupations into two main groups: the childcare workers (those workers involved in the provision of childcare, especially for young children) and social care workers (those workers involved in the provision of social care for both adults and children). This method has been described more fully elsewhere (Simon and Owen 2005). This analysis has been updated for this book and refers to data from the 2001–2003 Labour Force Survey.

The Labour Force Survey (LFS) is the largest of the UK government's regular household surveys (Owen 1999). It is a national survey collecting data from approximately 60,000 private households per quarter. The survey is conducted by the Office for National Statistics (ONS); full details of the survey methodology are available in the *LFS User Guide* (Office for National Statistics 1999). The LFS provides information about occupations using the Standard Occupational Classification.

The analyses presented in this chapter refer to Great Britain. All population figures in the tables are population estimates. However, for some categories, the sample numbers for a single year may be too small for reliable estimates (e.g. men working in childcare). Therefore, data have been combined over three years: 2001, 2002 and 2003, in each case using data from the first quarter (March to May).[2] These figures are shown in tables 2.1–2.3. Table 2.1 shows the occupations that make up each of the two groups of formal workers, and the job titles used to identify the workers within these occupations. It is a workforce that amounts to just over 1 million workers: 307,000 childcare workers and, 839,000 social care workers.

Table 2.2 shows that the formal care workforce is stongly gendered being 88 per cent female (98 per cent of the childcare workers and 85 per cent of the social care workers). In contrast, 46 per cent of the whole workforce is female. These care workers are predominantly white (95 per cent of the childcare workers and 92 per cent of the social care workers), in line with the workforce as a whole (94 per cent). Childcare workers are younger than the average for the whole workforce, and social care workers are older: 53 per cent of childcare workers are aged 35 years and over compared with 70 per cent of the social care workers and 63 per cent of the whole work-force. Care workers are mostly married or cohabiting (65 per cent of both childcare workers and social care workers) and have very similar levels of qualifications, with 51 per cent of childcare workers and 61 per cent of social care workers qualified to NVQ level 3 or above. Perhaps reflecting the different age profiles of the groups, childcare workers are slightly more likely than social care workers to have resident children (51 per cent compared with 40 per cent); non-resident children are not asked about in the LFS. Both groups of workers are relatively poorly paid: the childcare workers earn on average £7,850 (€11,302[3]) per annum gross and the social care workers earn on average £11,672 (€16,805) per annum gross; this compares to an average gross annual income for all workers of £17,859 (€25,713).

Despite these broadly similar characteristics, there were some important differences between childcare and social care workers, for example in terms of hours worked and hourly pay (Table 2.3). In childcare, workers were employed for on average 29 hours per week, with a mean hourly rate of £5.59 (€8.05), whereas social care workers reported an average 32 hour working week, at a mean rate of £7.15 (€10.29) per hour. Levels of remuneration for both groups were lower than the average hourly rate for all workers, of £9.55 (€13.75), and were even low in comparison to all female workers, whose average pay was £8.24 (€11.86) per hour.

Social care workers were more likely to work full time (57 per cent) than childcare workers (51 per cent), and to have received education and/or training in their jobs during the past 13 weeks (46 per cent compared with 39 per cent of childcare workers). They were less likely to be employed by a private firm or business (40 per cent compared with 63 per cent of childcare workers). There were striking variations between public and private sector[4] workers in relation to their pay and working conditions. For instance, draw-ing on figures from the LFS again, childcare workers in the private sector earned an average of £4.64 (€6.68) per hour, compared with average hourly earnings of £6.10 (€8.78) for public sector childcare workers. Similar

Table 2.1 The formal workforce

Care workforce group	Occupations	SOC codes	Related job titles	Total numbers of workers (thousands)
Childcare workers	nursery nurses	6121	• nursery nurses • nursery assistants • senior nursery staff	136
	childminders etc.	6122	• childminders • nannies	113
	playgroup workers	6123	• playgroup/preschool workers • playgroup/preschool leaders • playworkers and play leaders	59
	Total childcare workers			307
Social care workers	social workers	2442	• child care officer • child protection officer • social worker • team leader	77
	youth and community workers	3231	• youth workers • community workers • family centre workers	73
	housing and welfare officers	3232	• advice worker • care officer • counsellor (welfare services) • education welfare officer • housing officer • welfare officer	117
	houseparents and residential wardens	6114	• houseparents (boarding schools, residential care) • residential wardens • foster carers	31
	care assistants and home carers	6115	• care assistant • home care assistant • night care assistant • residential social worker	541
	Total social care workers			839
	Total care workers			**1,147**

Table 2.2 Some characteristics of childcare workers and social care workers (%)

	Female	White	Aged 24 and under	Aged 35+	Below NVQ 2	NVQ 3 equivalent or above	Married or living with a partner	Co-resident children
Childcare workers								
Nursery nurses	99	95	33	44	20	46	58	43
Childminders etc.	98	94	18	57	22	26	65	53
Playgroup workers	94	94	16	67	22	39	80	69
Total	98	95	24	53	39	38	65	51
Social care workers								
Social workers	77	86	3	80	4	81	68	43
Youth and community workers	74	90	8	67	11	63	58	40
Housing and welfare officers	74	91	4	74	11	66	65	38
Houseparents and residential wardens	89	99	3	84	15	42	71	32
Care assistants and home carers	90	92	13	66	20	22	65	40
Total	85	92	10	70	41	37	65	40
All care workers								
Total	88	93	14	56	40	38	65	43

Table 2.3 Working conditions of childcare workers and social care workers

Occupations	Average gross annual pay	Total usual hours in main job	Average gross hourly pay	In permanent job (%)	Working for private firm or business (%)	Full-time in main job (%)	Received education and training in past 13 weeks (in work)
Childcare workers							
Nursery nurses	£9,328 €13,430	31	£5.94 €8.55	92	50	66	45
Childminders etc.	£7,158 €10,305	32	£4.64 €6.68	79	89	50	26
Playgroup workers	£5,204 €7,493	19	£5.54 €7.98	91	44	17	51
Total	£7,850 €11,302	29	£5.59 €8.05	89	63	51	39
Social care workers							
Social workers	£19,811 €28,524	36	£11.47 €16.51	90	6	75	57
Youth and community workers	£15,837 €22,802	33	£9.67 €13.92	81	11	63	57
Housing and welfare officers	£16,383 €23,588	34	£9.76 €14.05	88	13	72	51
Houseparents and residential wardens	£13,031 €18,761	45	£6.67 €9.60	96	38	83	50
Care assistants and home carers	£8,986 €12,938	31	£5.71 €8.22	94	55	50	42
Total	£11,672 €16,805	32	£7.15 €10.29	92	40	58	47
All care workers							
Total	£10,776 €15,515	32	£6.79 €9.78	91	46	56	45

cross-sectoral variation in pay was found in the social care workforce: private sector workers reported an average hourly rate of £6.85 (€9.86), compared with £8.44 (€12.15) per hour on average in the public sector.

Workers' characteristics also varied within each of the two main occupational groups. Within the field of childcare, the Standard Occupational Classification (Office for National Statistics 2000) distinguishes between nursery nurses, who care for children under five in settings such as day nurseries; playgroup workers who deliver and facilitate play opportunities for children (usually 3 to 4-year-olds) in formal and informal settings including playgroups, play schemes, free play locations and after school activities; and childminders and related occupations, who perform a variety of domestic activities in the day-to-day care of children.

As Table 2.2 shows, nursery nurses were younger than other childcare workers (33 per cent were aged 24 or under, compared with 16 per cent of playgroup workers and 18 per cent of the childminders). Given that playgroups tend to operate part-time, it is perhaps not surprising that playgroup workers were unlikely to work full time (17 per cent compared with 66 per cent of nursery nurses and 50 per cent of childminders). Childminders were the least qualified childcare workers (26 per cent have an NVQ level 3 or equivalent qualification, compared with 39 per cent of playgroup workers and 46 per cent of the nursery nurses), and the lowest paid, earning an average of £4.64 (€6.68) per hour, compared with £5.94 (€8.55) per hour for nursery nurses and £5.54 (€7.98) per hour for playgroup workers.

The Standard Occupational Classification (Office for National Statistics 2000) distinguishes between the following groups of social care workers: social workers, defined as those who provide information, advice and support to protect the welfare of (various) groups including children, young people, families and people with disabilities; houseparents and residential wardens, who are responsible for the care and supervision of children, young offenders and the elderly within residential homes, schools or institutions for young offenders; youth and community workers, who provide support to individuals or groups of individuals through activities or services that aim to encourage participation in social, political and community activities; care assistants and home carers, who attend to the personal needs and comforts of the elderly and infirm, within residential establishments or at home; and housing and welfare officers, whose role is to assess and address the housing needs of particular localities and individuals, assist people with disabilities, investigate cases of child neglect or ill treatment, 'and perform other welfare tasks not elsewhere classified' (Office for National Statistics 2000: 118).

In line with findings for childcare workers, there was notable variation between these categories of social care workers. Relative to other social care workers, those categorised as social workers and houseparents/residential wardens were slightly older (80 per cent of social workers and 84 per cent of houseparents and residential wardens were aged 35 years and over, compared with 67 per cent of youth and community workers, 74 per cent of housing and welfare officers, and 66 per cent of care assistants). Care assistants, and houseparents/residential wardens were more likely to describe themselves as 'white' than other occupational groups (90 per cent of care assistants and 89 per cent of houseparents and residential wardens, compared with 77 per cent of social workers, 74 per cent of youth and community workers, 74 per cent of housing and welfare officers). Care assistants and houseparents/residential wardens were also the least qualified of all social care workers (81 per cent of social workers, 63 per cent of youth and community workers and 66 per cent of housing and welfare officers were qualified to NVQ level 3 or equivalent, compared with 22 per cent of care assistants and 42 per cent of houseparents and residential wardens). Care assistants were also least likely to work full time (75 per cent of social workers, 63 per cent of youth and community workers, 72 per cent of housing and welfare officers and 83 per cent of houseparents and residential wardens worked full time, but only 50 per cent of care assistants did so) or to have received on-the-job training during the past 13 weeks (only 42 per cent of care assistants reported such training, in contrast to 57 per cent of social workers, 57 per cent of youth and community workers, 51 per cent of housing and welfare officers and 50 per cent of houseparents and residential wardens). Differences in pay within the sector corresponded to variation in workers' qualifications. The highest paid were social workers, youth and community workers and housing and welfare officers, with average hourly rates of £11.47 (€16.51), £9.67 (€13.92), and £9.76 (€14.05), respectively. This compares with houseparents and residential wardens, who reported average hourly pay of £6.67 (€9.60), and care assistants who earned on average just £5.71 (€8.22) per hour.

Informal care workers

In defining some care work as informal, we posit three key characteristics: the work is largely unpaid, it is not formally (externally) organised or regulated, and it consists of caring for a person or people with whom the carer has an existing relationship. Informal care work is thus often carried out within families, for example in the care of elderly parents, or partners, children or grandchildren, and other family members (Mooney et al. 2002). It also includes care provided for non-family members, such as that carried out by neighbours or for friends. According to the 2001 census, 'A person is a provider of unpaid care if they give any help or support to family members, friends, neighbours or others because of long-term physical or mental health or disability, or problems related to old age' (Office for National Statistics 2003b). As well as being unpaid, informal care work contrasts with formal employment in its lack of set working times or duration for the work, and the (often very close) personal relationship that the carer has with the person for whom they are providing care. Informal care work is often carried out in conjunction with some kind of other paid work, and consequently, it must be fitted in around any paid work duties.

The General Household Survey (GHS) of 1985 for the first time included a set of questions about informal care provision (Green 1988). The questions were repeated in 1990 and 2000, and the GHS is now the main source of national data on informal carers (Rickards 2004). According to the GHS for 2000 (Maher and Green 2002), one in six people in Britain aged 16 or over was caring for a sick, disabled or elderly person.[5] Women were more likely to be engaged in informal care (18 per cent of female respondents) than men (14 per cent), and were more likely than men to carry the main responsibility for caring (11 per cent of women and 7 per cent of men were the main carer). Just over half (52 per cent) of those with caring responsibilities were caring for a parent or parent-in-law; one-fifth (18 per cent) were caring for a spouse and a further 8 per cent were caring for their disabled or sick children. Further, more than a quarter of these carers spent at least 20 hours a week on caring, with women spending more time caring per week than men. The highest time commitment to caring was found when the carer lived in the same household as the person being cared for. A fifth of carers (21 per cent) had been looking after someone for at least ten years. One-fifth (21 per cent) of economically inactive respondents had caring responsibilities, compared with 13 per cent of full-time workers, 17 per cent of part-time workers and 15 per cent of the unemployed.

In 2001, the British census included for the first time questions from the GHS on caring responsibilities (distinct from paid employment) for family members, friends, neighbours or others because of long-term physical or mental ill-health or disability, or problems related to old age, and asked about time spent on caring in a typical week. The GHS includes more detail on caring responsibilities and a wider range of demographic information than the census. However, the great benefit of the census is that it includes all people, whereas the GHS consists of a sample of approximately 14,000 adults. The census thus allows more reliable estimates to be made for small groups, for which the sample size in the GHS would be too small to be reliable. Where they can be compared, the results from the GHS and the 2001 census are consistent.

The census found that there were 5.2 million carers in England and Wales, including over a million providing more than 50 hours a week of informal care (Office for National Statistics 2003a). Of the 15.2 million employees aged 16–74 in full-time work, 1.6 million were providing at least some unpaid care, of whom, 144,000 providing 50 or more hours a week. Nearly 80,000 people aged 54 or under, providing more than 50 hours of unpaid care per week, stated that their own general health was not good.

Some small-scale studies have also examined the extent and nature of informal caring. For example, Kodz et al. (1999) estimated that six million people in the UK (excluding parents caring for non-disabled children) do some informal caring; Joshi (1995) found that one in seven of the workforce in 1990 were involved in caregiving and Phillips (1999) estimated that as much as a third of any workforce will be carers. To illustrate the characteristics of this informal workforce, this chapter will draw on the recently completed 'Fifty Plus' study (Mooney et al. 2002) which incorporated an analysis of national employment statistics, a large-scale survey of employees, and in-depth interviews with both carers and non-carers. The present chapter will highlight findings from large-scale statistical analyses conducted as part of this research; a more detailed account of which is presented in chapter 9.

Analyses of national employment statistics (using data from the Labour Force Survey) indicated that growing numbers of women in their fifties and sixties lived in households where both partners work. Consequently, the provision of informal care is likely to involve more juggling of schedules and time commitments than would be the case if one partner was at home full time. This national picture is helpful in identifying who is potentially available to do the caring, and the amount of potentially available time that individuals (as well as families) have to carry out these informal care duties. However, that interpretation is based on an assumption that less formal working means greater availability for informal care. In fact, the Fifty Plus study showed families and individuals to be under increasing pressure to work longer hours and still carry out informal care.

The employee survey from the Fifty Plus study illustrated the characteristics of this informal workforce in terms of the average length of time spent on care work per week, the gender of the average carer, the average age of carers, the marital status of these carers, the family set-up of carers (own/ step children, grandchildren, whether carers parents/parents-in law are still alive), the occupational grouping of carers that were working (the proportions of carers in manual, semi-skilled, skilled, professional or managerial jobs that had caring responsibilities), and the amount of paid work being carried out by informal carers. Most of the results from this employee survey corresponded to findings from analysis of the General Household Survey. In particular, it was evident that women, rather than men, did most of the caring and that caring often took place in combination with some other, paid, employment.

Phillips et al. (2002) have also examined the experiences of working carers of older adults. These informal carers often had multiple caring roles, juggling work and the care of both adults and children. Very few carers lived with the people they cared for, although one in three lived close by (within a ten-minute drive). Two out of three carers in their study spent less than 10 hours per week looking after others. Help with shopping and transport, emotional support, and 'checking' on people were the most commonly performed tasks, with few working carers providing very 'heavy' personal or physical care.

Other care workers

As discussed earlier in this chapter, much care work today cannot be clearly categorised as formal or informal. Rather, it seems to cross-cut the definitions of the two previous groups, sharing features from both. For instance, the care work may be voluntary (and unpaid) but linked to some sort of formal organisation, or there may be a formal relationship between the person being cared for and the carer, as in the case of mentoring (see chapter 7) or the carer may not be formally employed, but nevertheless paid some fees or expenses (e.g. foster carers).

Volunteers working in social care offer our first example of these workers. They do not include paid workers employed by the voluntary organisations, but rather provide unpaid help to other individuals on a voluntary basis. They have their lack of payment in common with informal care providers, but perhaps have more similarities with formal care workers. For example, voluntary workers do not generally have a close personal relationship with the person or people for whom they provide care, and often their care work is linked to, and regulated by, a large formal organisation. Voluntary organisations may also use procedures similar to those used in formal employment, for example in recruiting, assessing and training potential workers.

Since 1997, the UK government has developed a number of policy initiatives which emphasise the role of the voluntary sector in public service provision (Kendall 2000). A recent Home Office survey of almost 15,000 adults living in England and Wales (Munton and Zurawan 2004) found that 28 per cent volunteered formally at least once a month, with 37 per cent reporting informal voluntary activity in the preceding month. Of those engaged in formal voluntary work, nearly one quarter (23 per cent) reported activities related to health, disability, or social welfare; 16 per cent described their field of interest as 'the elderly', and a further 26 per cent did voluntary work relating to out-of-school activities with children and young people. Without more detail of the voluntary work itself, it is not possible to judge what proportion of these voluntary workers were engaged in care work, rather than other activities such as fund raising. However, as an indication, 19 per cent of all those volunteering formally were involved in 'befriending or mentoring work'. Compared to figures for 2001, the survey indicated a growing proportion of adults doing voluntary work, although women describing their ethnicity as 'white' formed the largest proportion of formal (30 per cent) and informal (41 per cent) volunteers. This finding is consistent with the observations of Knapp et al. (1995) that mostly females are attracted to volunteering. These authors also noted that adults and retired people are more likely to volunteer than young people (peaking at middle age), that people of white ethnic origin are more likely to volunteer than those from minority ethnic backgrounds, and that people with greater educational attainments and higher incomes are more likely to volunteer.

Organisations in the voluntary sector often focus on a particular group, such as children, older people, or one-parent families, or on a particular issue such as drug dependency, homelessness or dementia. Examples of such organisations include Barnardos, Age Concern and the National Association for Care and Resettlement of Offenders (NACRO). Barnardos, for example, has a number of ways that volunteers can contribute to the organisation's work: helping as a shop assistant, a driver collecting donations, as an administrative assistant, as a fundraiser. These examples show that volunteers even in an organisation involved in care provision may not be involved in direct care. However, there are also roles for volunteers which involve direct support to the target group (for Barnardos, children), such as befriending young people at risk of going into care, befriending young people leaving care without the support of a family, and assisting care leavers to develop independence and become a positive part of their community.

Mentors provide another example of volunteers playing a part in the care workforce, sharing features of both formal and informal care work. Mentors are similar to the informal care workforce in that they are usually unpaid, they are not employees, and so do not have a formal job description. However, they have similarities with formal care workers: the working organisation for which they volunteer defines their role, and they may make a commitment to volunteer for specific amounts of time. In addition, they have a formally defined relationship with the client. In this case, their role is to work directly with young people deemed to be in need of some specific support, working alongside that young person towards achieving a pre-stated desired goal.

Chapter 7 draws on the interim findings from an evaluation of national mentoring programmes for the Youth Justice Board for England and Wales, to describe in detail mentors that work with young people at risk of offending. These mentors contribute in many ways – from befriending them and by talking and doing activities with young people such as the cinema, bowling and sports venues to helping them to improve their basic numeracy and literacy skills – all with the aim of trying to reduce the likelihood of the young person re-offending. The chapter argues that all volunteer mentors should receive some training to help them work directly with young people in this way, although only half of the mentors included in the evaluation had completed their training before being assigned a young person to mentor. The mentors involved in this research had usually been assigned a particular individual to work with for a set number of hours, and more than half (57 per cent) of the mentors were also in paid employment, either full-time or part-time. The average age of these mentors was 34 years; 66 per cent were female, and 63 per cent were 'white'. This percentage is much lower than for workers in other parts of the care workforce, both formal and informal, and can be explained by the mentoring projects' recruitment policies, which aimed to include a high proportion of mentors from a minority ethnic background.

For the purposes of the discussion presented here, foster carers can also be defined as other care workers. Foster care is a regulated work practice, the caring is for a young person not related to the carer, and the work is usually done for some sort of payment. These characteristics would seem to suggest that foster carers are formal care workers. However, the fee paid to foster carers potentially has two components: an element to cover the expenses incurred in looking after the child, and an element of reward. Only the 'reward' element is taxable. Each year, the Fostering Network publishes its estimate of the weekly costs of fostering a child, according to geographical location and the age of the child. In 2004, these allowances ranged from £108.49 (€156.20) for a child aged under five years out of London to £224.50 (€323.23) for a young person aged 16 and over in Inner London (Fostering Network 2005). Nevertheless, the Fostering Network has shown repeatedly that the majority of local authorities do not even pay enough to cover the actual costs, quite aside from any element of 'reward', so that most foster carers are arguably receiving no pay for their work (Fostering Network 2003). Foster carers therefore have a lack of financial remuneration in common with informal care workers. The growth in kinship care also has similarities with informal care work. Increasingly foster carers are caring for relatives and others already known to them: in 2003, 18 per cent of foster placements in England were with relatives or friends (Department for Education and Skills 2004a).

In terms of demographic characteristics, Bebbington and Miles (1990) defined the archetype foster family as consisting of two adults, only one of whom was in full-time employment, with children of their own but none under the age of five, with a mother between the ages of 31 and 55, and living in a home with three or more bedrooms. The Berridge report (Berridge 1997) highlighted in addition the limited availability of foster carers from minority ethnic backgrounds. More recently, Triseliotis et al. (2000) confirmed these patterns. They found that 99 per cent of foster carers in their study described themselves as white, that only 8 per cent of fostering households had no children of their own, that four-fifths of carers were living with partners, mostly married and seven out of ten carers owned their homes with no more than three bedrooms. They also found similar patterns of employment for foster carers – 72 per cent of men and 37 per cent of female carers were in employment, and 60 per cent of the employed female carers were in part-time employment.

However, some men contribute equally with their partners to the provision of foster care (Sellick and Connolly 2001) and there has been a rise in the proportion of minority ethnic carers (Sinclair et al. 2000). Indeed, even Triseliotis et al. noted that only 35 per cent of foster carers fit the traditional image of the woman caring for the children at home while the man provides the family income outside the home. Like the other care workers in this group, female foster carers are increasingly seeking employment in addition to the care activities they are carrying out, and much of this paid work is within the social care sector: around two-fifths of female carers had a social care sector job, including childminding and nursery work (Triseliotis et al. 2000).

Conclusions

In this chapter, we have drawn a practical distinction between two forms of care worker: the formal and the informal. The formal care workforce is defined by its constituent occupations: these workers are paid for the care work they do, they may be required to have some degree of formal training, and they are regulated in what they do. At the opposite end of the spectrum, we have situated the informal workforce. These care workers have little or no formal recognition for the work they do, no requirement for formal or informal training, and they often provide care work in addition to other paid work. We have also argued that other workers, such as volunteers and foster carers, share qualities of both formal and informal care.

In describing the characteristics of formal, informal and other care workers, the chapter has highlighted undeniable differences between the three workforces, but also a number of important similarities. Shared characteristics include gender (more females than males in each case), age (people of 'middling age' are most attracted to the work, although, as we have discussed earlier, childcare workers, and particularly nursery workers, are relatively young care workers). Arguably, these groups of workers might also share common values, underpinning their motivation to participate in what is often low paid or unpaid work, an issue that will be illuminated by the contrasting discussions of different forms of care worker in chapters 6 to 9.

Government policy places great emphasis on the importance of volunteering and its role in citizenship (Kendall 2000; Popple and Redmond 2000), but it has been argued that changes in the voluntary sector are in danger of squeezing out the volunteer – 'the new climate of contracts and professionalisation will result in a squeezing out of volunteers altogether, or at least a fundamental shift in the values and culture of volunteering' (Commission on the Future of the Voluntary Sector 1996). At the same time, there are dangers in assuming that the voluntary sector offers low cost means of service provision, given evidence of the costs and organisational demands of reliance on a volunteer workforce (e.g. McGonigle 2002).

With the costs of social care escalating as the UK struggles to cope with an ageing population, the government has emphasised the need for families to provide more of the care themselves. In England, a National Strategy for Carers (Department of Health 1999) has recently been published. In a forward to the strategy the prime minister, Tony Blair, says, 'we all may need care, or to provide care ... Carers will have better information. They will be better supported. They will be cared for better themselves. What carers do should be properly recognised, and properly supported – and the government should play its part' (Department of Health 1999: 3–4). The strategy includes proposals to increase the carers allowance by an extra £50 (€70) a week in real terms by 2050, schemes to help carers to return to work, better information for carers about the health of the person they are caring for and how to cope with that, support for neighbourhood services such as carers' centres and special funding for breaks for carers.

This chapter has also highlighted the common experiences of different parts of this care workforce, for example, relating to lack of payment of informal and some other care workers, such as volunteers. As one example, the variations in the payment of expenses between local authorities is said to have led many foster carers to leave the public sector altogether, or to move into the independent sector. According to one local authority manager of social care services for children and families, 'In the first five months of this year alone, the council has seen 10 of its 100 carers leave and move across to the private sector to be employed by independent fostering agencies (IFAs)' (Community Care 2003). According to this article, it is not only the lack of basic expenses payments that has led to this crisis, but also the lack of support and perceived value of foster carers' work.

There has been some movement towards procuring greater value from the care work for the carer themselves. For instance, voluntary work can offer a potentially flexible means for those with other commitments, such as work or family responsibilities, to gain training and experience that could create future opportunities for paid employment. This benefit has, however, con-comitant organisational implications (and costs) relating to turnover of voluntary workers.

In summary, the discussion presented here illustrates the inter-relatedness of formal, informal and other care workers, and, as noted earlier, these are not mutually exclusive categories, but rather a useful definitional rubric for analysing the field. As subsequent chapters in this volume illustrate, these forms of care work each have a role to play in future developments, and they are clearly envisaged as doing so in English policy today. For example, unpaid informal or voluntary workers may be seen as offering a partial solution to cost concerns, or to staff shortages in the formal workforce. And, just as the formal/paid workforce recruits workers from the 'in-between' workforce in times of shortage, the 'in-between' workforce may recruit workers from the formal/paid workforce to meet shortfalls in supply (Boddy et al. 2004). The care workforce may be unusual, in relation to other sectors of work, in that it relies on a substantial component of informal workers to address shortfalls in the supply of formal paid workers. That said, questions remain about how far the different groups of workers are equivalent, and the remainder of the book will highlight these issues – for example, with regard to the need for a professional knowledge base for care, or the particular values that underpin unpaid work such as mentoring.

Our distinction between formal, informal and other care workers is argu-ably artificial, but provides a necessarily practical means for determining 'who are today's care workers', in terms of the specific occupations that underpin the formal care workforce and the characteristics of those carrying out care work. However, the analysis has not addressed the inter-relatedness of different elements of the care workforce, or the movement into, out of and between care occupations, or of how different forms of care work might interact over the life course. This chapter has made use of a number of statistical data sources, which may focus on different aspects of care. The proposal for the Office of National Statistics to combine its five major household surveys into one survey (Office for National Statistics 2004) may make it easier in the future to get a more joined-up picture from a single source.

Notes

1   Data for Northern Ireland are not included in this chapter.
2   Material from the Labour Force Survey is Crown Copyright, has been made available by the Office for National Statistics (ONS) through the UK Data Archive and has been used with permission. Neither the ONS nor the Data Archive bear any responsibility for the analysis or interpretation of the data reported here.
3   An exchange rate of £0.69455 per euro has been used. This was the exchange rate quoted by the European Central Bank on 27 October 2004: http://www.ecb.int/stats/exchange/eurofxref/html/index.en.html
4   Definitions are taken from the Labour Force User Guide (April 2003): the private sector consists of all private firms or businesses or limited companies, and public companies (plc); the public sector is defined as being comprised of nationalised industries/state corporations, central government, civil service, armed forces, local government or council, universities, polytechnics, other grant funded educational establishments, health authorities or NHS trusts, charities, voluntary organizations or trusts, and 'other' organisations (ibid.: 69).
5   These only include children if they fall under the criteria of sick or disabled. All other forms of childcare are not included here.

3 Nineteenth-century understandings of care work

Pat Petrie

Introduction

Historical sources provide a means of examining the present in light thrown from times past: looking at how things *were* can cause us to question how things *are* and bring us to a greater realisation that many of the concepts we turn to frequently today are historically specific to our own age. While many of today's social programmes and provision have developed to meet current concerns, within a specific national, political and historic frame-work, they also have roots in the past. This chapter examines care and care work as we perceive these phenomena today, in their nineteenth-century manifestations.

The understandings we bring to history grow out of present-day concerns and theoretical perspectives. The chapter will take as its starting point some of the main areas and themes arising from today's theorising of care. They are themes that are discussed throughout this book: the gendering of care work, issues of social class, questions of training and qualification, the location of care and provision in the private and in the public sector, the ethos of care, the work involved in caring, and care as responsibility. These are themes and areas that intertwine.

The chapter will mainly draw on nineteenth-century evidence, because it was in this century that public welfare policy, as we know it in the United Kingdom today, developed and expanded. Although there had been statutory support for the poor since Elizabethan times, and a much longer history of charitable support, both of these expanded in the nineteenth century. Social and economic forces – 'improved' farming and the development of industrial mass production accompanied by financial speculation – had brought labourers into the towns. Compared to their earlier position, poor people were now highly visible, they could be seen *en masse*, their extreme poverty, ignorance and 'vice' became offensive and had to be addressed by new, or improved, public measures: the movement for popular education is a prime example (Petrie 2003). Among those who sought to influence these measures were politicians, novelists, philanthropists, and the early social scientists.

At the same time as the development of public welfare policy, including the early development of the regulation and inspection of provision, the nineteenth century was to see a growing consolidation of occupations that relate to care work in our own century. This chapter will bring together a range of occupations that today are referred to as caring, social care and care work. And, in the nineteenth century as today, they were occupations that might be paid or unpaid, undertaken on the basis of private relationships and responsibilities, or on the basis of professional and employed status. They covered the care of the poor, of children, of the sick and the elderly infirm. They took place in the carer's own home, or in that of the person cared for, and in a wide range of institutions. For the purposes of this chapter, notions of care will be expanded to take in the related occupations of teaching and nursing. The boundaries between care and each of these two occupations were, as we shall see, sometimes clear, sometimes blurred – just as they have continued to be in recent times.

Why fiction?

Novels offer one arena for an historical exploration of care and care work, alongside other documents and histories. They colour our imagination and underpin some of our understandings, while at the same time they can challenge common assumptions about how things were in the past. So this chapter will use nineteenth-century novels as sites for an historical exploration of care and care work, alongside other documents and histories. This is not to claim that novels represent 'truth' or 'reality': they are of course fictions coloured by their authors' understandings and values. Nevertheless, novels furnish common reference points for the consideration of times past. They provide more subjectively based insights into the ethical climate of their time than do many other social documents. Novels can show how things work out for individuals and can help us to understand more vividly the social contexts for care, and the conflicts of interest that care work involves. Because fiction can illuminate other historical sources and, in turn, be illuminated by them, the chapter also draws on non-fictional records.

Some of the novels upon which the chapter is based are qualitatively different from many of those published today. They were not only about personal life but aimed at contributing to public debate and political decisions. Many nineteenth-century novels were widely distributed, and read not only as a private but as a communal pleasure: they were read aloud and shared. They were, therefore, especially available for forming a common mind. They could be influential in shaping the perceptions, both of the general public, and of that section of it which was socially powerful. Many of the novelists to whom we shall turn led a public as well as a private life, they were well informed on social matters and brought to them a powerful, philanthropic analysis. For example, Dickens remained a working journalist throughout most of his writing life. In writing many of his novels, his intentions were explicitly didactic and political. He researched his work, often had personal experience of the conditions about which he wrote and he aimed at reform. Similarly with the novelist Elizabeth Gaskell, who as the wife of a non-conformist clergyman in the north of England saw for herself the injustices, misery and hypocrisy of industrialised society. Anthony Trollope was in rather a different position, in that he decried the campaigning methods of Dickens (whom he pilloried as 'Mr Popular Sentiment' (Trollope 1925: 203, Chapter 15, first published in 1855). He, like Dickens, led a public life. As a civil servant, travelling the country, he was in a position to understand and comment on the ethics of public and commercial office, the subject of many of his novels.[1]

There are many contemporary non-fictional accounts that attest, explicitly, the veracity of the social understandings displayed in nineteenth-century fiction. Thomas ('Dr') Barnardo, describing, not care work, but destitute children in London, said:

> We also thought that the stories about their conditions and suffering in London which have attracted attention were mainly furnished by the vivid imaginations of certain writers whose love for the sensational had overcome their strict regard for the truth. That this is the state of mind felt by a very large number of persons, we feel assured, although they . . . have never yet been brought face to face with these awful facts in our social history, which however much they may appal and shock, must nevertheless be admitted as true.
>
> (writing in *The Christian* 22 August 1872,
> quoted in Wagner 1979: 31)

In the preface to the first complete edition of *Nicholas Nickleby* (Dickens Undated (a): xvii, in serial form, from 1839), Dickens wrote that several headmasters had recognised themselves in the portrait of a brutal head-master, Squeers, and been affronted by it. He said, however, that 'Mr Squeers is the representative of a class and not of an individual' (ibid.). Squeers operated within the private for-profit care market – although it was not so named at the time. His Yorkshire boarding school took in unwanted boys, such as disabled children, step-children and 'natural' sons, whose parents wished them to be in the care of others, far from their own homes.

Dickens noted that 'Mr Squeers and his school are faint and feeble pictures of an existing reality, purposely subdued . . . lest they should be deemed impossible' and in a preface to *Nicholas Nickleby* (ibid.: xix) said that at the time of the first publication (that is when it had appeared as a serial) there were 'a good many cheap Yorkshire schools in existence. There are very few now', implying that the novel had played its part in exposing them and leading to their demise. (His part in this demise was also believed by other commentators; see, for example, Hammerton Undated: 218; Miltoun 1904).

Ethics of care

Dickens' portrayal of the Yorkshire schoolmasters was fuelled by anger. Having roundly condemned the 'monstrous neglect of education in England' that allowed them to function without any qualification, he continues

> Traders in the avarice, the indifference or imbecility of parents and the helplessness of children; ignorant sordid brutal men, to whom few considerate persons would have entrusted the board and lodgings of a horse or a dog; they form the corner-stone of a structure which, for absurdity and a magnificent *laissez-aller* neglect, has rarely been exceeded in the world.
>
> (Dickens Undated (a): xx)

The anger that blazes through this passage stems from an ethical base: the schools manifest venality and they are a travesty of care. Uncaring carers, carers who are 'on the make', with no regard for those in their care, are the frequent objects of Dicken's anger: Mrs Gamp, the squalid nurse in *Martin Chuzzlewit* (Dickens Undated (b) First published in book form 1844), and Mrs Mann and Mr Bumble in *Oliver Twist* (Dickens Undated (c); serialised from 1839) who care nothing for their charges, but much for their own social aspirations and the accumulation of wealth, come readily to mind. They helped form some public perceptions of what we now see as care work, and perhaps they still do.

Clearly the ethical dimension of care has long been recognised. More recently, Joan Tronto (1993) has written that the ethic of care is about practice, and ways of perceiving what should be done for others and with others, rather than about applying rules or principles. This view of ethics focuses on relationships and empathy with the 'other', it belongs to the realms of feelings and of conscience more than to philosophy and logic: it is territory that is home ground for the novelist.

In the nineteenth century, the ethical dimension of care was seen as both connected to principles of obligation and duty,[2] and to personal relationships, warmth and devoted practice. A computer search of the texts of *Nicholas Nickleby* and of *David Copperfield* (Dickens Undated (d); serialised from 1849) finds frequent reference to care in the sense of principles of obligation and duty.[3] For example, a cold and calculating brother-in-law (Ralph in *Nicholas Nickleby*) speaks of his obligations to his brother's widow and daughter: 'Your mother and sister, sir . . . will be provided for . . . by me, and placed in some sphere of life in which they will be able to be independent. That will be my immediate care . . .' (Dickens Undated (a): 28, Chapter 3). Ralph is portrayed as having no feelings of empathy towards his relatives, and only reluctantly assuming the 'care' which would be expected of him – that which, in fact, transpired to be a minimal, and conditional, financial support.

In both novels, care as duty owed to another is also, on occasion, coupled with notions of warmth and affection, of duty and work undertaken in such a way that they speak of fellow feeling. A passage from *Nicholas Nickleby* speaks of Newman Nogg's immediate physical work on behalf of his friends (as do other incidents in the novel): 'There was a fire in Newman's garret, and a candle had been left burning; the floor was cleanly swept . . . meat and drink were placed in order on the table. Everything bespoke the affectionate care and attention of Newman Noggs' (Dickens Undated (a): 416, Chapter 31). In *David Copperfield*, a woman speaks of her father: 'I have always aspired, if I could have released him from the toils in which he was held, to render back some little portion of the love and care I owe him, and to devote my life to him' (Dickens Undated (d): 776, Chapter 54). Here, duty and love seem to go hand in hand.

These examples depict care as an aspect of private relationships. But there are also fictional examples of caring where people are paid to take responsibility for others. In Trollope's *The Warden* (1925 first published in 1855), the Reverend Septimus Harding is in charge of an almshouse for old men. He relates to them individually and personally, and is devoted to them. The author commented:

> . . . they have warm houses, good clothes, plentiful diet, and rest after a life of labour; and above all that treasure, so inestimable in declining years, a true and kind friend to listen to their sorrows, watch over their sickness, and administer comforts as regards this world, and the world to come!
>
> (Trollope 1925: 43, Chapter 4)

Harding loses his post as warden and is succeeded by a steward, who is not personally involved with his charges, who takes care of the physical maintenance of the buildings, but nothing else: he has no 'care' in any sense of that word for the almsmen (Trollope 1925: 275, Chapter 21). The steward is not portrayed as at all villainous, unlike Squeers, but he is a paid official for whom any ethical standards connected with care, or duty, do not involve personal relationships.

Harding received a stipend for performing his duties. Caring responsibilities of many sorts were also undertaken on an unpaid basis and are portrayed as either virtuous, when conducted with empathy and unmotivated by self-interest, or as interfering and callous, when undertaken in a spirit of self-aggrandisement. Much has been written concerning the particular feminisation of women, as 'angels in the home' during the nineteenth century, and how the emotional spheres became increasingly polarised between the private, domestic, caring and personal (feminine) and the public, impersonal and more 'manly' emotions. This is an area needing further exploration, which we return to in greater detail, below.

In Elizabeth Gaskell's *Ruth* (1967, first published in 1853), an unmarried mother, the daughter of a farmer, is taken with her illegitimate baby into the household of a dissenting minister as an act of uncondescending, and courageous, care – even though the minister prompts Ruth to assume the identity of a widow. The novel makes plain the hypocrisy of the double standards of the time, by which upper-class men may, without opprobrium, seduce lower-class women, who are then outcast from respectable society. The novel was deeply controversial in its subject matter and in its judgements. Elizabeth Gaskell, against the prevailing ethos, conveys, with understanding, the circumstances that led to Ruth becoming an unmarried mother: her lack of family and material support, her youth and ignorance of sex, and her high-spirited readiness to enjoy life. But these alone were far from enough to mitigate Ruth's 'sin' in the eyes of the reading public. Her innate goodness had to be made apparent through her actions. Ruth's redemption lies in her virtuous care of her son, her care as portrayed in her role as governess to a local family and finally, during a typhoid epidemic, in her becoming an unpaid 'matron' in the local infirmary, nursing the dying poor, before going on to nurse the man who had seduced her. She is held before the reader for admiration and compassion. 'Few were aware of how much Ruth had done; she never spoke of it, shrinking with sweet shyness from over-much allusion to her own work at all times' (ibid.: 425–426, Chapter 33). Ruth's own resulting death may be seen as restoring the virtuous femininity of a 'fallen' woman or, perhaps even for Gaskell herself, Ruth's sacrificial works are evidence of her redemption: 'it was she who had gone voluntarily, and with no thought of greed or gain, right into the very jaws of the fierce disease' (ibid.: 426 Chapter, 33).

In *David Copperfield*, (Dickens Undated (d)) we meet Little Em'ly, another 'ruined' woman, for whom Dickens demands our sympathetic understanding. He also legitimises the readers' sympathy for her by showing her, at the end of the novel, as a caring woman. Her uncle tells of their voyage to Australia: 'But theer was some poor folks aboard as had illness among 'em, and she took care of *them*; and theer was the children in our company, and she took care of *them*; and so she got to be busy, and to be doing good, and that helped her . . . [She was] fond of going any distance fur to teach a child, or fur to tend a sick person' (ibid.: 868–869, Chapter 63).

For both of these fictitious women, Ruth and Little Em'ly, their authors see teaching and looking after children, and care for the sick as related activities – 'womanly' work, when accomplished selflessly and with sensitivity.

On the other hand, voluntary activities undertaken without any fellow feeling were open to criticism. In *Bleak House* (Dickens Undated (e) serialised from 1852), we meet the formidably busy Mrs Jellaby: 'The African project at present employs my whole time. It involves me in correspondence with public bodies, and with private individuals anxious for the welfare of their species all over the country. I am happy to say it is advancing' (ibid.: 38, Chapter 4). Dickens despises and lampoons this character – perhaps more especially because she addresses her good cause at the expense of her own children. In the same novel, Mrs Pardiggle, whom the author treats with an even colder disdain, is accompanied, unwillingly, by her five sons, on various self-assumed duties: 'I am a School lady, a Visiting lady, I am a Reading lady, I am a Distributing lady; I am on the local Linen Box Committee, and many general Committees . . .' (ibid.: 103, Chapter 8). The reader is shown her in action, haranguing a brickmaker, in his squalid hovel, while his wife nurses a dying baby, before our eyes (ibid.: 109). There follows an immediate comparison with the empathetic care shown by another, poor, woman. The story's narrator comments, 'I thought it very touching to see these two women, coarse and shabby and beaten, so united; to see what they could be to one another; to see how they felt for one another . . .' (ibid.: 111). For this novelist, social class alone does not qualify a person to take charge of the welfare of others: the ethical dimension is also important.

Questions of qualification, employment and social class

Part of Dickens' critique of Jellaby and Pardiggle is that they are 'unfeminine', as evidenced by the uncaring neglect of their own children. In lampooning them, he invites contempt for all such publicly active women. Yet women's public activities were often uniquely important, as the work of many Victorian female reformers testifies. In addition, public work could give middle- and upper-class women occupations to fill their time, and provide interests that were sometimes passionate. With housework performed by servants, and childcare by nannies and governesses, these women had time on their hands. But, not only were they unqualified for paid employment, to undertake such work was almost unthinkable. The father of Sophia Jex-Blake, the pioneer of women as doctors, told her that if she accepted a salary she 'would be considered mean and illiberal . . . accepting wages that belonged to a class beneath you in social rank' (Peterson 1972: 5). It was unacceptable for unmarried middle-class women to undertake paid employment, other than to be a governess (see below), and for a married woman to do so was quite unthinkable. Voluntary work would thus seem to be the only path open, whether caring morally and physically for the poor, or organising means to further their welfare.

Mrs Jellaby and Mrs Pardiggle had no specialist qualification for the work which they undertook, and the same was true for Mr Harding. In the nineteenth century, to belong to the respectable classes was often itself sufficient qualification for the oversight of, and responsibility for, other people. Unless experience proved otherwise, a person who belonged to the respectable classes was perceived as being of good character, their religious affiliation was taken for granted and they would have, at least, some 'appropriate' level of education. The opposite held true for those who were not respectable: the indigent and, probably criminal, poor. For example, because Mr Harding was a clergyman, he was seen as ethically 'sound' and his appointment as warden was therefore appropriate – even though his honour might be (in the novel it was) called into question. He was also a person of education, in that he had taken a university degree, a customary qualification for membership of the clergy. Trollope's pastiche of a pamphlet directed against Harding, says: 'our modern friend shall be a man educated in all seemly knowledge: he shall, in short, be that blessed being – a clergyman of the Church of England' (1925: 196, Chapter 15). Trollope is not well disposed towards Harding's detractors, but the ironic tone of the passage reveals that the right of the clergy to take on roles by reason of their office was not without challenge.

In the social world, as opposed to the world of fiction, religious affiliation could also be as important as a qualification for undertaking care work. For example, Thomas Barnardo sought to employ 'Christian housewives' as housemothers to take charge of cottage homes for destitute children and, in another case, a 'Godly brother' and his wife were employed to be the resident governors of a home. (Wagner 1979: 79, 52). Such men and women might not share the social status of Harding, Pardiggle and Jellaby, but they were drawn from the respectable working classes and their adherence to Christianity (and perhaps especially the enthusiastic evangelism espoused by Barnardo) appeared to fit them for the residential care of children.

Similarly, inherent qualities perceived to adhere to social class qualified the governess and the tutor for their work. Tutors and governesses were seen as sufficiently qualified by their own, middle-class, education and moral values, to take on the education and daily care of children and young people. The male tutor's initial education was 'higher' than that of women, because they either had a degree or at least had received something of a classical education – the education of 'gentlemen'. Nevertheless, it appears that not all tutors had a degree. Nicholas Nickleby (Dickens Undated (a)) was an exploited teacher, in Dotheboys Hall, the school owned by Squeers. Nicholas had left school at around the age of 18, on his father's death, without going on to university. Forced to earn his living, he applied for the job of master at Dotheboys Hall, although he did not have the MA that its advertisement would have, disingenuously, 'preferred'. While his work encompassed education (of a sort), it also contained what would now be seen as 'care work'. For example:

> a few slovenly lessons were performed, and Squeers retired to his fireside, leaving Nicholas to take care of the boys in the school-room, which was very cold, and where a meal of bread and cheese was served out shortly after dark.
>
> (ibid.: 97, Chapter 8)

Had he the qualification afforded by a degree, Nicholas could have sought a more favourable position, perhaps one in which education played a much larger role relative to that of care and surveillance. Indeed, later in the novel, he tries his hand at such a position, as a visiting (non-resident) tutor in a private household.

The governess, too, performed a role that was both caring and educational in that it required her to protect, oversee and teach children. This was in accordance with the understanding that any middle-class woman was fitted to bring up children and to provide an appropriate education for girls, and young boys. But, whether she herself had been taught at school or in her own home, there was no guarantee that she was fitted to educate others. 'The most noteworthy feature of middle class girls' education in the first half of the 19th century was its variability' (Gorham 1982: 21).

Nineteenth-century literature provides a great many examples of men and women who turned to becoming governesses and tutors because they could not afford to live independently and needed food, shelter and a small salary. In 1850 there were some 21,000 governesses, whose status was insecure and whose salary was low (Hollis 1979: 48). Governesses, in fiction, ranged from the amoral Becky Sharpe in Thackery's (Undated) *Vanity Fair* (an exploiter, rather than herself exploited), to the near saintly Jane Eyre (Brontë 1953, first published in 1847). For Gwendolen Harleth in *Daniel Deronda* (Eliot 1984, first published in 1876) becoming a governess was abhorrent. Her impoverished mother learns of a possible position for her in a bishop's family and tells her, 'your French, and music, and dancing – and then your manners and habits as a lady, are exactly what is wanted . . .' Gwendolen replies, 'Excuse me, mamma. There are hardships everywhere for governesses. And I don't see that it would be pleasanter to be looked down on in a bishop's family than in any other' (ibid.: 199). Eventually Gwendolen chooses a loveless marriage, rather than submit to such social stigma. The governess, and indeed the tutor, inhabited a no-man's land between the family and the servants, belonging to neither one group nor the other. In *Jane Eyre*, Jane is maliciously subjected to a long-winded belittling of governesses by the guests of her employer: 'I have just one word to say of the whole tribe; they are a nuisance,' says Blanche Ingram to her mother and to the general company (Brontë *op. cit.*: 176, Chapter 17).

To some extent, the governess was worse off than the tutor. Because she lacked the liberal education of her male counterpart, which might include a university degree, she had less power and was more open to exploitation. Hence her position was especially marginalised and badly paid. Nevertheless the governess avoided 'the immodest and unladylike position of public occupation' (Peterson 1972: 6). However destitute, a governess was, by definition, a 'lady', and this was her qualification for looking after the children of other ladies and gentlemen. The exploitation of governesses took place within the private domain of the home, or the private school. They – unlike trained nurses, who favoured private nursing (see below) – were unqualified and untrained.

Public disquiet on behalf of governesses was such that a benevolent association was set up on their behalf, drawing, no doubt, on the energies of activists like Mrs Jellaby, and of other more likeable ladies. This association was formed in recognition that some of the problems inherent in the position of the governess arose because they were neither properly prepared nor qualified for their role. So, the association set about educating girls:

> Queen's College was opened on the 1st May, 1848. It was an offshoot from the Governesses Benevolent Institution; which is a society having for its design to benefit an important and very interesting class of our country women, not only by affording assistance to them when in difficulty, sickness and old age, but by raising the standard of their accomplishments and thus entitling them to higher remuneration.
> (*Queen's College Quarterly Review* 1850, quoted in Hollis 1979: 136)

Bedford College, a similar institution, was to follow.

As today, issues of qualification, gender and social class intertwined. The genteel education of young ladies, and the liberal, classical education of their brothers, was the private responsibility of their parents, although it was often accomplished by others. However, during the nineteenth century the state assumed responsibility for a more utilitarian, instrumental education – elementary education for the lower classes, which eventually became universal and free.[4] Elementary school teaching did not recruit ladies, but rather the daughters of the skilled working classes. After an apprenticeship, working-class young women went to teacher training colleges to prepare for work in the public elementary school (Burdett-Coutts 1979: 91). Once trained, these women obtained better pay and a more secure livelihood than was the case for many governesses. Their favoured position was the result of acquired, rather than ascribed characteristics, and they were qualified through study rather than through their social origins. Women teachers were socially upwardly mobile. This alarmed some members of the upper classes, who thought that their training and quasi-professional occupation ill-suited them for their eventual role as wives and mothers, who would need to perform the mundane work of domestic care. However, Dorothea Beale – a pioneer in the education of middle-class girls – thought highly of the elementary teachers and employed them because they were better teachers than the unqualified middle-class governesses, asking 'How is it that the daughters of the higher middle class are more ignorant and untrained than the children of the national schools?' (Beale 1865, quoted in Hollis 1979: 137). At the same time, she realised that they were unskilled in accomplishments such as French and music – the domain of the governesses – and so additional staff were required for these specialisms.

While middle-class girls appeared to their employees as fitted by nature and upbringing to become governesses, and the daughters of artisans could train to be teachers, poorer working-class women were fitted, it seemed, for more lowly paid care work. They needed no training and could even perform the work alongside other domestic tasks, as part of the normal role of working-class women. Mrs Betty Hidgen, in Dicken's *Our Mutual Friend* (Dickens Undated (f) serialised from 1864), is a fiercely independent washer-woman and childminder (in today's jargon, a 'family day care worker'). All her life, she says, she has 'worked when she could, and she starved when she must' (ibid.: 206, Chapter 16). Aged nearer to eighty than seventy, she keeps her charges sitting under the clothes mangle, as she works, and explains 'I keep a Minding-School. I can only take three, on account of the mangle. But I love children, and Four-pence a week is Four-pence' (ibid.: 205, Chapter 16). She is also, in some sense, a foster carer for Sloppy, a 'love child' sent to her by the poorhouse, who now turns the mangle. The extract reminds us of how close personal and domestic service is to care work. A family is cared for via traditionally maternal, domestic tasks: cooking, shopping, washing, cleaning and 'minding' children. These tasks are seen as coming naturally to Mrs Higden: as a respectable working-class woman, she has been brought up to them and no qualifications are necessary.

Mrs Higden works in her own home. Other working-class women per-formed care work in other people's homes. In Martin Chuzzlewit, Mrs Gamp's 'profession', as Dickens refers to it, is to be 'a nurse and watcher, and performer of nameless offices on the persons of the dead' (Dickens Undated (b): 322, Chapter 19); she is also a midwife. All these nursing tasks were performed, as was usual, without qualification. The portrayal is in part comic – she is one of Dicken's grotesques, drunken, dishonest and on the make – but it also provides an example of callous disregard and lack of care for those she is supposed to ensure are 'carefully looked to' (ibid.: 432, Chapter 26). Mrs Gamp is also paid for her work, unlike little Em'ly or Ruth (see above).

Mrs Gamp worked privately, but until Florence Nightingale introduced training, nurses working in public hospitals were also untrained. The follow-ing extract from Elizabeth Garrett, writing in the Transactions of the National Association for the Promotion of Social Science, in 1866, makes the social class basis of different forms of care work clear, and also links care work to personal service and domestic work. Of the head nurses, she says:

> As a rule they are skilful experienced and kindly people, very well-suited to the work. They usually belong to the lower section of the middle-class, are the widows of small tradesmen or clerks, or less frequently they have been confidential domestic servants . . . The under nurses wait upon the patients, assist the sister in her duties, and in many cases clean the wards . . . They are commonly below the class of second or even third-rate domestic servants: if they were not nurses, one would expect them to be maids of all work, scrubs or charwomen . . . From them, again, there is an apparent descent to the night nurses . . . when they do not live in a hospital, they eke out their scanty incomes by working the best part of the day, and consequently they come to hospital hoping to be able to sleep the better part of the night . . .
>
> (quoted in Hollis 1979: 96)

Even after Nightingale introduced training, many trained nurses preferred to work in private homes,[5] rather than look after poor people in the public infirmaries or, worse still, in the workhouses, where trained nurses were rare.

Gender and care

Men have been precluded, over the last century, from many forms of care work, whether public or private. It is tempting to see current movements towards sexual equality in caring as progressing from a time when there was even greater gender differentiation. As we have seen, for the Victorians being a carer was linked to roles construed as feminine: the care of the sick, the upbringing and education of children. Sensitivity, kindness and nurturance were seen as coming 'naturally' to women, and associated with notions of the ideal women; a prime example is contained in *The Angel in the House*, a sequence of poems by Coventry Patmore, written between 1854 and 1863 (Patmore 1998).[6] But we should not, therefore, think that men were complete strangers to care work and caring. In the nineteenth century, gender differentiation in these areas was not clear cut. Both fictional and historical accounts indicate that men had a place in the Victorian world of care and care work which needs to be distinguished and acknowledged.

In Victorian novels, we find male characters portrayed as carers, in the sense that they take on personal care work. They are as devoted to those for whom they care as many women characters who appear in the same works. Their authors do not depict them as unusual, *as men*, for undertaking these duties – although they are portrayed as admirable *human beings*.

In the case of Mr Harding, in Trollope's *The Warden* he is depicted as devoted to the old almsmen, he gave them comfort, companionship and support, and sat with them when they were ill. Turning to care at the other end of the life cycle, Silas Marner (Eliot 1996, first published in 1861) is no stranger to childcare. He had looked after his little sister 'whom he had carried about in his arms for a year before she died, when he was a small boy' (ibid.: 110–111, Chapter 12). When he takes in an abandoned toddler, Eppie, her (undisclosed) biological father comments, 'that's strange for a miser like him' (ibid.: 118, Chapter 13), but the strangeness is located in Marner's character, rather than his gender.

With high levels of maternal mortality, many widowed men must have found themselves looking after their children. This is not to say that the women in *Silas Marner* see the men as adept as themselves. Neighbours wonder how Marner will manage with a 2-year-old child on his hands (ibid.: 120, Chapter 14). Others remark that Marner is 'partly as handy as a woman' (ibid.: 130), while his principal adviser observes, 'I've seen men as are wonderful handy with children. The men are awk'ard and contrairy mostly, God help 'em, but when the drink's out of 'em they aren't unsensible' (ibid.: 122). Marner's care of, and for, Eppie are the making of him. From being a crabbed miser, he becomes a warm, happy and well-loved step-father, respected in his community. While caring for others seems to restore femininity to Ruth and Em'ly (above), for Marner it appears to give him back his humanity.

A commentator (Christ 1977: 160) draws attention to men who take on a nurturing role in nineteenth-century literature. She discusses what she calls 'Dicken's preference for older, essentially motherlike men', who look after children, care for the sick and helpless 'in ways that are self abnegating and essentially feminine'. She holds that many Victorian writers desire to incorporate feminine qualities in men in order to counterbalance prevailing images of masculine aggression. However, caring is not confined to Dicken's elderly men. A striking example of a young male carer is Nicholas Nickleby, who physically cares for the delicate Smike, not only during a long journey from Yorkshire to London, but also during his final illness.

> By night and day, at all times and seasons, always watchful, attentive, solicitous, and never varying in the discharge of his self-imposed duty to one so friendless and helpless as he whose sands of life were now fast-running out and dwindling rapidly away, he was ever at his side. He never left him; to encourage and animate him, administer to his wants, support and cheer him to the utmost of his power, was now his constant and unceasing occupation.
>
> (Dickens Undated (a): 773, Chapter 58)

That men looked after and nursed other men, in private, should not be surprising – they were certainly to be found in the public sphere. In the workhouses, on male wards, elderly men were to be found as nurses. Frances Power Cobbe, writing in 1861, observed:

> In the male wards they are usually old men . . . in the women's the most depraved and abandoned. The ways in which a hard unfeeling nurse may torment her wretched patient are beyond enumeration.
>
> (quoted in Hollis 1979: 249)

In the navy and army, especially, men were required to look after each other.[7] Men cared for the sick or wounded on board ship – the surgeon's mate would be seen as a theatre nurse today – but others did the lower level tasks involved in the care of their wounded shipmates. In naval hospitals, until 1883, nursing was undertaken by men, who were:

> usually ex-seamen or marines, who were recruited as required from the shore establishments and who held no nursing qualifications. An earlier experiment to introduce female nursing had generally proved unsuccess-ful and unpopular, though a few female nurses were still employed.
>
> (National Archives Research Guides 2004b)

Men were also nurses in field hospitals in the army. Indeed, with the Nightingale reforms and the gradual professionalisation of nursing, the army initially set its face against employing trained women as nurses – not least because they were outside the military chain of command and thus somewhat independent. Nightingale, for her part, was opposed to men in nursing and promoted the idea that to be a 'good nurse' was also to be a 'good woman'. Male nurses in workhouses, field hospitals and on board ship had not trained as nurses, but learned, or failed to learn, on the job – just as untrained women did in a variety of care settings.

Brown et al. (2000) have commented on the feminised nature of nursing that emerged in the nineteenth century, suggesting that the earliest nurses were men and that references to support this are to be found in the earliest Hippocratic writings. They say, 'nursing is unique in that during the late nineteenth century it became an almost completely "feminised" occupation, following what Theweleit calls a "new female assault" on medical and caring work. Before this, women did little more than midwifery' (Brown et al. 2000: 1). These authors discuss nineteenth-century changes in the constructions of masculinity, describing how in the early part of the century, men had more physically intimate attitudes to friendship and to caring. These were re-worked over the course of the century, resulting in the avoidance of sensitivity, nurturance and emotion as defining masculine characteristics.

Victorian and other literature provides many examples of men displaying tender emotions, and it is well documented that politicians sometimes wept in the course of delivering an impassioned speech. Clearly, the relationship between gender and caring has a complex history, and we cannot assume that twentieth-century stereotypes have always held sway.

Messages from the past

We can see from nineteenth-century fiction that, although the term 'care work' was not in use, care and caring were powerful concepts, just as they are today. In depicting Sarah Gamp, Betty Higden, Ruth, Wackford Squeers, Septimus Harding and Jane Eyre, the novelists allow readers to glimpse something of the lived experience of caring and being cared for nearly two centuries ago. Caring and being cared for were intimately bound up with birth, life, death, love and well-being, and betrayals of care were betrayals of other, more vulnerable, people. Then, as now, caring was seen as an activity that could be judged on moral, as well as practical, dimensions. Care work is not merely the domain of mundane activities. Overseeing children's meals or sitting up with the sick are certainly means of earning a living – or at least of getting by – but they are also human activities, based on relationships between people, rather than a series of robotic or technical actions.

While people who cared for others were, then as now, in a position of trust, they could also themselves be vulnerable; carers may exploit and/or be exploited. Both caring and the employment of carers are ethical matters, as the novels that this chapter has glanced at vividly reflect. The role of the carer can have much in common with that of the servant, in that it is based on an unequal relationship favouring the 'master', or employer, especially in labour markets where unskilled people need work. The nineteenth century saw the beginnings of the professionalisation of teaching and nursing, reducing the vulnerability of people in these occupations. Training for governesses was introduced in order to strengthen their social position, as well as enhancing their own education.

Care and care work are the products of specific social contexts. In the nineteenth century, just as people had multiple social positions (for example, they were poor or rich, men or women, married or not, belonging to the respectable or to the indigent classes), so their 'caring' roles differed: the jobs that they undertook, their qualifications, whether they worked in the public or the private sphere were all linked to social standings that had more than one dimension. Caring and care work related, and continue to relate to governing ideologies: to being feminised or masculinised in ways that adapt to other social conditions, and to the governance of the workforce in the ways that support current concerns for economic growth, social stability and (in the nineteenth century) the maintenance of empire:

> What reason perceives as its necessity, or rather, what different forms of rationality offer as their necessary being, can perfectly well be shown to have a history; and the network of contingencies from which it emerges can be traced. Which is not to say, however, that these forms of rationality were irrational. It means that they reside on a base of human practice and human history; and that since these things have been made, they can be unmade, as long as we know how it was that they were made.
>
> (Foucalt 1988: 36–37)

The intention of this chapter has been to illuminate some of the processes inherent in care and care work. In the nineteenth century, a newly industrialised society saw change and development, with care becoming more formalised, more subject to qualification and (although we have not touched on this) to legislation and bureaucracy. There was, as we have seen, something of a movement from a society where it was acceptable for men to care and to show their emotions, to one where it was less so. Today, we have a technologically based society, with globalisation and an increased international movement of peoples: the social contexts for people's lives, from the family to the labour market, from schools to childcare, to hospitals, are also changing. For example, there has been some shift in the relative social position of men and women; in the minority world, migrant workers provide a new pool of labour; new forms of mass media both reflect and produce new consciousnesses of what it is to be human – to be young, to be old, to be sick, to be poor or to be rich. All of these factors affect what in this book we are calling care and care work, but they do not provide the entire picture. It is nevertheless possible to make collective judgements and take social decisions that shape society in one way or another (as a cross-national comparison of different types of welfare regimes reveals). The ethical dimension of care, with its basis in human relationships and social justice, was important for many of our nineteenth-century predecessors: it is no less called for in shaping the future of care and care work, today.

Notes

1 Anthony Trollope's mother, Fanny Trollope, also wrote many novels, whose subjects included social reform, child labour and the abolition of slavery.
2 Interestingly, a 'sinecure' means holding a job without any actual cares, i.e. duties.
3 It also occurs more colloquially, meaning being 'careless' about appearance, or not 'caring' to do something, meaning not wanting to do something.
4 'By 1861 women were 80,000 of the country's 110,000 teachers; by 1901, 172,000 out of 230,000, of which perhaps half were fully-trained and certificated, and earning around 75 per cent of the male rate. It was one of the few jobs that could be combined with family life, though men teachers made determined efforts to exclude women from the work' (Hollis 1979: 48).
5 One of the biggest drains on the pool of trained nurses were the 'private' or domestic nursing agencies who provided nurses for the care of the well-to-do in their own homes (National Archives 2004a).
6 Harriet Matineau's had been a nineteenth-century voice raised against Gaskell's *Ruth*, not because the novel was immoral, but because of what she saw as the timidity of the author (Uglow 1993: 342). Virginia Woolf, in 1931, was to speak in a lecture of the need for women writers to 'kill the Angel in the House' (Woolf 1970).
7 On board ship, the wives of non-commissioned officers also did nursing and other care work, just as in the army, the so-called 'camp followers' took on nursing and other care for soldiers.

4 Knowledge and education for care workers

What do they need to know?

Claire Cameron and Janet Boddy

In paid care work, issues of knowledge and education, and of their measurement through qualifications and training, are a definitional mine-field. One way of conceptualising knowledge is as a continuum (Greenwood 1957) from, at one end, concrete, specific and discrete items of information, and, at the other, generalised and theoretical systems, with all other knowledge between these two poles. The distinction between 'education' and 'training' is also not easy to make. For example, 'education' might refer to school, college or university-based courses and qualifications; 'training' to the workplace; and 'learning by doing', including competence-based qualifications emphasising a rather practical way of transferring knowledge. For the purposes of this chapter, however, we use 'education' as a generic term for the acquisition or construction of knowledge.

In this chapter, we contrast different approaches to knowledge and education – in particular what we shall term 'vocational-industrial education' and 'professional education' – drawing on cross-sectoral and cross-national research recently conducted at the Thomas Coram Research Unit, including a study of six countries called 'Care Work in Europe' (see Appendix for a research summary of this study). In particular, we shall compare three sectors in the UK, childcare, residential care for children and young people, and care for older people or social care.[1] Work in these sectors in the UK has long struggled with professional status. So for example, residential child care work, also known as residential social work, has been considered lower status than field social work and the expectation that staff hold qualifications has been lower than those for field social workers. Similarly, care work with elderly people is perhaps one of the lowest status social care occupations and has the one of the lowest levels of requirement for qualifications.

We also make a number of cross-national comparisons – in particular between care work with older people in England and with young children in Denmark – which illustrate how great the difference is between the two approaches and raise questions about the rationale for these national and sectoral differences. This contrast can be seen as representing two extremes of a continuum of requirements for formal education and raises some questions about the place of alternative kinds of knowledge.

A final point by way of introduction is to draw attention to a theme that runs through the chapter: the close relationship between the knowledge and education that are considered necessary and desirable for care work and how the work itself is conceptualised, including the social image of the group receiving care and what the care worker is expected to do. If the work is conceptualised as the performance of instrumental tasks in conformity to laid-down procedures, the kind of knowledge required is different to that where the care work is conceptualised as working with and through relationships, making finely tuned and contextualised judgements. It is also closely concerned with the question of professionalisation, as a developed and coherent knowledge base is arguably, or has been historically, a prerequisite for professional status.

Knowledge and education in care work today

The regulation of qualifications for care work

Since the 1980s, education and qualification for care work occupations in the UK has taken place through what might be termed an industrial-vocational system of workplace-based competency awards linked to the award of Scottish or National Vocational Qualifications (S/NVQs). Care work is viewed as an industry, or a number of industries, whose employees need to achieve industry-defined National Occupational Standards, which are statements of the skills, knowledge and understanding required in a particular industry and clearly define the criteria for assessing competent performance (Qualifications and Curriculum Authority 2004). In this system, employees' competencies are assessed in the workplace against a nationally recognised benchmark, with clear statements of required occupational performance, and with a continual assessment process that can provide immediate and frequent feedback to candidates (Sargeant 2000). As we will see later in the chapter, this contrasts with the approach adopted in some other countries where care work is conceptualised differently, and the implications for the knowledge and skills, and so the education required, may be different.

Within the UK system, qualifications are awarded at various levels ranging from Level 2, broadly equivalent to a school leaving qualification for a 16-year-old, to Level 5, equivalent to a higher education degree. The issue, therefore, is not just the approach adopted but the level at which qualifications for care work – or indeed any occupation – are pitched. None of the occupations considered here – residential social workers, day nursery workers, childminders, care assistants and home care workers, covering work with young children, social care work with young people and with older people – actually require a qualification in order to practise in the UK, at least in a non-managerial role. In other words, it is possible in the UK today to practise paid care work without any formal preparation by way of further or higher education. That said, for all groups there are national minimum targets in place to increase the proportion of the workforce that holds relevant qualifications. Table 4.1 compares these qualification targets for England, and the extent to which they have been achieved across the occupational groups.

Day nursery workers and childminders (family day carers) represent just two of the many occupations and job titles that describe those who work with young children in childcare services in England. Regulations stipulate that employers in day nurseries must ensure that the manager and supervisors hold a Level 3 qualification, that is, one designed for work without supervision, and at an upper secondary level (that is broadly equivalent to the school qualification of an 18-year-old); while half of the remaining childcare staff should have a Level 2 qualification, a low level of qualification where supervision is still required (Office for Standards in Education 2001a). The remaining staff need have no qualification at all. Childminders do not need formal qualifications to practise, but should complete a short local authority approved pre-registration course and a first aid course within

Table 4.1 A comparison of care occupations and the qualifications required, coverage, sector location and body responsible for qualifications: England

	Regulations – minimum qualification requirements	*Coverage in the workforce*
Day nursery workers	Managers and supervisors to hold Level 3*; 50% remaining staff to hold Level 2	50% Level 3 (mostly managers and supervisors); 20% no qualification
Childminders	No formal qualifications; Complete local authority approved pre-registration course and first aid course within six months of starting; be a 'suitable person'	64% any relevant training; 16% Level 3
Residential care workers	80% to hold Level 3 (by 2005)	33% estimated to achieve NVQ3 2002–2003 (public sector)
Home carers	50% to hold Level 2 (by 2008)	70% of providers have fewer than 20% staff with any relevant qualification
Care assistants	50% to hold Level 2 (by 2005)	70% of care homes employ staff group where fewer than 20% hold any relevant qualification

Sources: Department of Health 2002b, 2003a, 2003b; Eborall 2003; Office for Standards in Education 2001a, 2001b.

* Levels refer to NVQ levels: Level 2 is designed for occupations where supervision is required and is broadly equivalent to the English GCSE; Level 3 is designed for working without supervision and broadly equivalent to English A Levels.

six months of beginning work. The childminder should also be a 'suitable person', and have appropriate experience, skills and ability to look after children (Office for Standards in Education 2001b).

There is an incentive for nursery workers to obtain an education and a relevant qualification as their employment prospects are greater. As well as working in day nurseries, many work alongside teachers in primary schools, and prefer to do so because of better pay and conditions (Cameron et al. 2001), or as assistants in health settings or as nannies. For those intending to work as a childminder, there is no similar incentive: their life experience will qualify them adequately.

National regulations concerning education and qualifications for childcare workers were first introduced comparatively recently, under the Children Act 1989. One reason for this historic lack of attention to education for childcare work may be hinted at in the phrase 'suitable person', which dates back to early regulations on childcare providers (in legislation enacted in 1872 and 1948) and reflects an association between care for children outside the domestic home and experience of mothering (Cameron 1999; Hevey and Curtis 1996). This absence of national attention to education and qualifications for childcare workers, combined with practice recognition of the need for formal education, led to the development of substantial numbers of often local courses, many of which had little national currency, as will be discussed below.

There are far fewer residential care workers than childcare workers, as there are only about 7,700 children and young people in residential care in England. This latter figure includes accommodation in secure units, children's homes, hostels and residential schools. Residential care workers (also known as residential social workers and residential child care workers) do not have their own professional qualification in England. However, national regulatory standards, which cover children's homes accounting for 5,900 children (Department for Education and Skills 2003), required managers of residential homes to ensure that a minimum of 80 per cent of their care staff held a competency based award at Level 3 by January 2005 (Department of Health 2002a), which covers such topics as 'contributing to the protection of children from abuse; contributing to the development, provision and review of care programmes, and how to establish, sustain and disengage from relationships with clients'.

Historically, residential care has been linked to social work education, although, more recently, the relationship between the fields has become weaker, and has been the subject of some dispute. Milham and colleagues (1980) questioned whether residential care was 'like' social work, and so whether the training should be the same. In some respects, the work was distinctive – for example the group work dimensions of residential care, and the close proximity to the task – and these elements were not covered on social work courses. But in attempting to define the residential care workers' role, Davison (1995: 50) argued that many of its ethical principles were 'not dissimilar' to social work or 'people work' in general, and that the work was about 'providing young people with both the means and the opportunity for living a meaningful life, ensuring there is access to appropriate and effective help'.

In the late 1940s, a Central Training Council was set up to establish education for what were then known as 'housemothers' in residential care, which evolved into a Certificate in Social Service (CSS), a parallel qualification to the Certificate in Qualification in Social Work (CQSW) for field social workers. In 1990, the two certificates were replaced by the Diploma in Social Work (DipSW), and in 1992 the then social work education body, the Central Council for Education and Training in Social Work, set quality standards for residential care work, recommending that all such workers should hold a professional qualification at DipSW level (Heron and Chakrabarti 2002).

In the early 1990s, a secondment drive led to many residential care workers completing the DipSW. However, on completion many became field social workers, where the status and pay were better, leaving residential care again with unqualified recruits (Community Care 2003). Meanwhile, social work became a three-year (Level 5) degree course in 2003, but the main qualification for residential care work was, and is now, established as an industrial-vocational and competency based (Level 3) S/NVQ. While this distinction appears striking, Jones (1996) argued that the DipSW demands and curriculum have become ever more prescribed, so the distinction between the two forms of qualification may be more imaginary than real. Similarly, Heron and Chakrabarti (2002) have contended that both the DipSw and NVQs are competence based.

Of the three types of care work discussed here, education for care work with elderly people is least developed; the main occupations are domiciliary or home care work (home carers) and institutional-based residential care work (care assistants). Historically, home care work in the UK was defined as domestic assistance (Sinclair et al. 2000), but has shifted towards health tasks and personal care in a policy era that has emphasised care of elderly people in their own homes and communities (Department of Health 1998). Care assistants have similarly faced a gradual change of role, towards caring for more severely disabled elderly people than used to be the case (Johansson and Moss 2004).

As with other care work occupations, national standards have been introduced. Each residential home manager must ensure that at least half the care staff held a NVQ Level 2 qualification by 2005 (excluding any nurses) (Department of Health 2003a); and 50 per cent of home care workers are similarly required to hold NVQ Level 2 awards, but by 2008 (Department of Health 2003a). The emphasis is on showing that staff are 'competent and trained to undertake the activities for which they are employed and responsible' (Department of Health 2003a: Standard 20.1). But as with childcare work, this standard means that up to half the staff will not be required to have any specialist education by way of preparation.

Vocational qualifications (S/NVQs) are intimately linked to national occupational standards and so are rooted in practice requirements, rather than education in a wider sense, and the appropriateness of competence-based vocational qualifications for care work has been subject to some debate. A study of the impact of S/NVQs on residential child care workers found that all respondents had had negative experiences: they had not learned new things; they felt their writing skills were assessed rather than their practice; there was excessive repetition, confusing jargon that was irrelevant to practice; and successful completion depended to a great extent on the assessor and workplace support available, which was variable. Positive effects were limited to increased awareness of their practice through doing the NVQ, although this could lead to spending work time looking for items to use as evidence rather than actually being with the young people (Heron and Chakrabarti 2002).

By contrast, a larger scale survey of social care staff working across residential day and domiciliary care found several benefits associated with NVQ training. These included workers' improved performance, which was sustained over time, increased appreciation of and willingness to promote the concept of good practice, heightened awareness of their own limitations and training development needs; respondents also rated NVQ training more highly than other forms of training (Sargeant 2000).

The extent of qualification in the workforce

Regulatory requirements for qualification levels are only one influence on UK education in care work. Despite the rather low regulatory requirements, education for childcare workers has proceeded apace through local recognition of the benefits of education for work with young children. An audit in 1998 found that 329 specific qualifications were recognised as suitable by regulating authorities in the UK, half of which were national programmes and half were locally available courses such as pre-registration courses for childminders (Cordeaux et al. 1999). Attempts to rationalise this multiplicity have been made through the introduction of a national framework of 'early years education, childcare and playwork' qualifications (Quality and Curriculum Authority 1999). Pathways from childcare work to teaching and management have also been developed through foundation degrees, early childhood degrees, masters' degrees in early childhood studies, and leadership programmes.

However, childcare workers are poorly qualified compared to the female population overall, and most of the qualifications held are of the industrial-vocational variety. As Table 4.1 shows, about half of day nursery childcare staff hold a Level 3 qualification, mostly concentrated among senior managers and supervisors, while 20 per cent do not hold any qualification at all

(Surestart 2004). Among childminders, levels of education and training have been increasing rapidly, despite the lack of formal requirements: 21 per cent held any relevant qualification in the late 1990s (Mooney et al. 2001), rising to 64 per cent in 2003, although only a sixth (16 per cent) held at least a Level 3 childcare relevant qualification (Surestart 2004). Recent policy efforts in England to raise the quality of childcare services have included the education of childminders through the establishment of childminder networks. Through membership of such networks, a childminder can be accredited to offer early education to 3- and 4-year-olds. Eligible childminders have to be approved using a quality assurance scheme and, through the network, take part in ongoing monitoring and training to support the educational part of their work.

Studies of residential care in the 1990s found that relatively few of the staff held a relevant qualification (Berridge and Brodie 1997). Given the complexity of work in this field, arguably its workers should receive an education to equip them accordingly. However, one study found that holding a qualification (which could come from many different fields such as social work, nursing, teaching, childcare) in itself was not a predictor of good outcomes for young people: more important was good leadership (Sinclair and Gibbs 1998). Having a coherent, single professional qualification for residential care may go some way to addressing this apparent discrepancy (Cameron 2004). Despite evidence of the role complexity in residential care, the policy shift has been to prescriptive, competency-based awards, which rely on assessors in workplaces to judge them. The regulatory requirements appear to be having some impact on workforce qualifications, although in 2002–3 qualification levels were well short of the target: only 33 per cent of local authority residential child care workers in England were estimated to have achieved Level 3, while no information was available on qualifications of staff in the independent sector (Eborall 2003).

The 'Social Pedagogy Study' (Petrie et al. forthcoming), found that English residential care staff in the public and private sectors were less likely to hold a qualification (and where they did it was less likely to be a 'high' level qualification) than their colleagues in Denmark and Germany. Moreover, when these staff were interviewed about ongoing training, respondents in England were less likely to have taken part in in-house training or training leading to a qualification than their cross-national colleagues and were more likely to say they had done an 'other short course' (for further details see chapter 6).

The concept of a preparatory knowledge base of any kind is far from established in care work with elderly people. There is some evidence that home care workers are reluctant to complete formal training programmes due to their age or believing it is unnecessary for their work, although many believe there are benefits to clients from having trained staff (Francis and Netten 2003). In a survey in England in 2001, nearly three-quarters of (70 per cent) of care homes were recorded as having fewer than a fifth of staff holding any relevant qualification, and as even fewer managers hold qualifications (Eborall 2003) there is little 'lead from the top' on developing a knowledge base. In home-based care a similar situation pertains; in 2001, 70 per cent of providers had fewer than a fifth of employees holding a relevant qualification (Eborall 2003). Moreover, relatively few domiciliary care providers were enrolling their workers in NVQ programmes: three-quarters had fewer than 20 per cent of staff currently undertaking NVQs at the time of the survey (Eborall 2003). Achieving an improved knowledge base in care work with elderly people is under severe challenge from simul-taneous policy drives to casualise the work, which erodes conditions of work and encourages a transient workforce (Eborall and Garmeson 2001).

Sector location and its impact on qualification levels

Most care work in the UK is now located in the private sector (see chapter 2), mostly in for-profit provision. Childminding has always been a private-sector occupation, albeit with varying levels of public-sector support. Similarly, nearly all the growth in day nursery provision since the mid 1980s has been in the private sector (Department for Education and Skills 2001b); although since 1997 substantial public money has been available to support the development of centres in socially disadvantaged areas, much of this provi-sion is located in the private sector. Since the 1980s there has been a major ebbing of residential and home care from the public to the private sectors (Eborall 2003), and a similar trend, although it occurred later and to a less significant degree, can be seen in the management of children's homes (Commission for Social Care Inspection 2004).

Simon et al. (2003) have reported that sector location has an impact on pay: private sector social care and care workers are paid less than those working in the public sector. Far less is known about the impact on uptake and completion of qualifications (Eborall 2003). In the 1990s, the private care home sector 'struggled to gain serious recognition of its commitment to training' (Godfrey 2000: 57), and preferred to focus on practical skills train-ing rather than 'higher level' qualifications. Early evidence, however, sug-gested that NVQ registrations were more common in the private and health sectors than in the local authority social services sector (Godfrey 2000), but more recently the private sector was reported to be less positive than the public sector about its ability to achieve the targets for NVQ qualifications among care workers (Eborall 2003). Demand was said to outstrip supply, there was a shortage of personnel for assessment purposes, and access to funding was complex (Eborall 2003).

Central concepts in qualifications for care work

In England, the central concepts in education to work with young children appear to be: recognition of relevant experience, which may be familial, domestic or voluntary, through the idea of assessing competency; practical and personal orientation to work and to education for work, through the idea of rewarding experience; and mastery of procedures through close linking of training to national occupational standards. Some criticism has been raised that childcare students on further education courses such as the Diploma in Childcare and Education, rather than following the NVQ route, are not learning to think critically but to perform in an imitative fashion (Alexander 2002). As Moyles (2001) argued, to think is to challenge, and there is a critical element in being a professional, whereas many early years workers are both motivated by their personal experience and at the same time are distrustful of and underestimate the value of their insights.

At present, there appear to be three main themes in education for work with young children in England: an unresolved debate about the values and purposes of childcare and early years services with a policy push for 'education' into 'care' services; minimal requirements for qualifications and low levels of qualification among the workforce; and attempts to address issues of raising quality through 'equalising' early years workers, so that accredited and networked childminders can offer the 'same' education as a nursery teacher can in a nursery or primary school. Alongside the push for early education, childcare workers are increasingly being relied upon to observe children's development and detect abnormalities. There is some evidence that early years and childcare workers are ill-prepared for this role and require more specialist training, for example in order not to miss children with speech and language difficulties (Mroz and Hall 2003).

Whether well-qualified individuals can raise the overall standards in a team environment is also open to question. Moyles (2001: 86) found that 'qualified teachers in the early years sector tend to work "down" to the level of their variously trained colleagues rather than raising the standards within their settings through acknowledgement of different roles, experience and expertise'. Sylva and her colleagues (2003), by contrast, found that having qualified trained teachers working with children for a substantial proportion of the children's time had the most significant impact on the quality of the service: less well qualified staff (mainly childcare workers) worked to a higher level when they worked with qualified teachers.

Residential care for children and young people had its early origins in replacement parenting and equipping young people with skills for work (institutions were called industrial schools and training schools in the nineteenth century) but, in the post-war era, became associated with the more treatment-oriented ethos of social work. There has remained confusion over the role of residential care; whether it is therapeutic, or is merely engaged in management or containment of young people's behaviour until their eventual 'release'. As if reflecting a move towards a procedural orientation to residential care, the knowledge base has now been firmly aligned in policy with the industrial-vocational type of competency award represented by the NVQ. Recent comparative research (Social Pedagogy 2) found that relative to Danish and German practice, English residential care workers were more reliant on procedures than other approaches to dealing with practice situations (Petrie et al., forthcoming), an issue discussed further in chapter 6. The question posed by Milham et al. (1980) and more recently reiterated by Smith (2003) remains: does residential care have its own values and purposes and ways of working and therefore require a distinctive knowledge base?

Research on work with elderly people has also found evidence of its complexity, requiring attention to detail, observational and reporting skills, and working with social relations, including sometimes delicate negotiations over daily life (Johansson and Moss 2004; Neysmith and Aronson 1996). A study of professional and moral development for care work with people with dementia found that while care workers often viewed situations with ageist assumptions and prescriptive solutions, through training and discussion it became clear that the task is more complex: 'not to make decisions for other people but to enrich and catalyse their decision-making' (Kitwood 1998: 405). With depth of knowledge about individuals, gained through introducing new responsibilities to learn about clients' histories, care workers in this study developed a 'richer compassion' for clients' lives and a greater respect for their care needs. The author argued that a 'good care worker should be able to act fluently, spontaneously, using his or her feelings and intuitions, combining a heightened sensitivity with mundane practical skill' (Kitwood 1998: 408). Each worker also has to optimise the well-being of all members of the group, and this can produce tensions in care workers' daily lives.

This study illustrates both the complexity of care work with demented elderly people and some ways in which the work can be transformed from the performance of physical tasks to relational work, through a focus on quality and reconceptualisation of the staff role. In this case it may be that the qualifications target of Level 2, although thought to be difficult to achieve, has been pitched too low to equate with the knowledge and skills required to care effectively for older people (Eborall 2003).

What knowledge is important for care work?

Three types of knowledge for care work emerge from this discussion, each of which is connected to how the care worker is conceptualised and what education is deemed necessary. First, there is *tacit knowledge* or practice wisdom, derived from personal qualities and experience, including as an informal or unpaid carer for family members. Tacit knowledge is the 'implicit store of knowledge used in practice . . . [and] is a meaningful and important source of information that influences practitioners' decisions and actions' (Zeira and Rosen 2000: 104). Wærness (1984) has argued that care work expertise derives from the carer's practical experience and personal knowledge of the care recipient; one has to understand from the position of an insider rather than rely on generalised scientific knowledge. This form of knowledge is arguably difficult to articulate and thus to evaluate (Wærness 1984), although Gustavsson (1996) argued that inability to articulate practice wisdom might in fact conceal a lack of knowledge.

Second, there is what might be termed *functional knowledge*, central to what we have termed the industrial-vocational approach to education and qualification. This approach to knowledge, focused on the ability to perform certain tasks to agreed standards, appears to predominate in the current English drive to 'upskill' the care workforce through industrial-vocational awards that show competence. Competence is incontestably desirable as a practice minimum: but might also be seen as anti-developmental in a peda-gogic sense (Smith 2003). Moreover, the relationship between qualifications for an occupation laid down in regulatory regimes and the knowledge and skills thought important to do the job is not necessarily straightforward; the former may be set at a level considered achievable by the 'care industry' overall, rather than at a level commensurate to the complexity and demands of the work.

The third approach can be termed *professional knowledge*, combining professional skills (including specific competences) and practical experience with a strong theoretical underpinning, and usually based in an academic setting (university or specialist college). Important here is the ability to relate these areas of knowledge – experience, skills and theory – especially through reflection. There are different views about the relative balance of theoretical education, practical experience and professional skills. For example, in a study of the education of nursery workers for the Care Work in Europe project, practice placements accounted for 13 per cent of course time in Spain but one-third in Denmark and Hungary (36 per cent and 33 per cent respectively) (Korintus and Moss 2003). Respondents involved in education argued that an adequate balance of theory and practice elements is import-ant to ensure that, as one said: 'theory feeds practice, but practice should feed back into theory. If there isn't a contrast, theory remains dead' (ibid.).

Although we have defined types of knowledge, we have also suggested that they are not necessarily mutually exclusive; indeed, a key issue is how the relationship between them is conceptualised and developed through educa-tion. Similarly, the location of education does not necessarily equate with a particular type of knowledge. University-based courses may be more or less prescriptive and focused on particular competencies, while workplace-based education may involve the development of professional knowledge with a strong emphasis on the relationship between theory and practice (see, for example, Rinaldi 2005).

A European comparison

Using data from two case studies conducted for Care Work in Europe, and in particular interviews with care workers, this section will discuss these ways of approaching knowledge and education contrasting two sectors and two countries – elder care in England (Cameron and Phillips 2003) and childcare in Denmark (Jensen and Hansen 2003). These two countries illustrate very different approaches to knowledge and education in care work: functional and industrial-vocational in England, professional in Denmark. However, even in Denmark, education and qualification for work with older people is less well developed than work with children, a feature of care work across Europe.

Sweden has the highest level of education for workers with older people, having moved from an initial reliance on 'housewifely competence' in the immediate post-war years to recognition of the need for formal education. The main occupation in this area of care work is the auxiliary nurse (*under-sköterska*), qualification for which requires three years, study at an upper secondary level (equivalent to the UK Level 3) (Johansson and Moss 2004). Establishing a commitment to an occupation and a knowledge base does not in itself ensure success: in the Swedish case, many courses have unfilled places and many who complete the courses go on to choose other fields of work or study, the auxiliary nurse qualification being recognised in other fields of work including in services for young adults with severe disabilities. In consequence, there are still a substantial number of Swedish eldercare workers who have not trained as an auxiliary nurse. Moreover, although the qualification level aspired to in eldercare in Sweden is considerably higher than in the UK, it is still below the achieved level in Swedish childcare services, which have been redefined as educational services: half of all workers are graduates, the remainder having an upper secondary qualification (Cohen et al. 2004).

Care work with older people in England

The case study of care work with older people involved interviews with policy-makers, trainers and sixteen care assistants and home care workers in rural and urban locations (Cameron and Phillips 2003). Care work informants indicated that they consider their jobs as involving both practical and emotional support, a combination of task-focused and relational work. As one informant, a home care worker, said:

> They are there for the clients to talk to, to confide in sometimes, you know, they need someone to confide in. People, they are kept clean, warm in their own homes, they have regular meals, and they are comfortable in their own homes.

Care work was seen as having an important benefit for relatives, who could share or be relieved of their informal care responsibilities, and for users or residents, who no longer had to cope alone. Having a formal service enabled elderly people to make choices about aspects of their lives, such as having a care worker to bathe them instead of a relative. It enabled social contact and reduced loneliness and could open up networks for older people.

These care workers thought others devalued their work, mostly perceiving it to be domestic tasks; many of the 'little personal things' they did for their clients went unrecognised. In residential care, the combination of tasks and relationships was also there, and the sense that 'you have to literally do everything for them up to what they require or what they'd like', but there was a greater sense of having to fit into a routine. With increased policy emphasis on independence and re-ablement through a 'National Service Framework for Older People' (Department of Health 2001a), some of the care workers in this study were aware that it was best to encourage users to do as much for themselves as possible (Cameron and Phillips 2003). One said: 'so long as they have got their independence to do it, I think it is nicer for them to be able to do it'. This shift reflects a change of philosophy within 'care': it is no longer caring to 'do things for' people; instead caring is observing what assistance people need, and providing it, to do things for themselves.

When it came to the knowledge and skills necessary to do care work, these care worker informants did not draw attention to changes in what they needed to know in order to adapt their working to the new policy emphases. Table 4.2 sets out their responses to a question about the knowledge and skills needed for care work with elderly people.

The knowledge and skills listed include personal skills such as respect, patience and intuition, and some workers directly attributed the knowledge base for their work to experiences of being a member of a family. Taught professional skills, such as observation and communication were also referred to. Two workers, both male, did mention formal knowledge such as health science and first aid as important for doing a good job in care work, though overall relatively little emphasis was placed on medical or social knowledge. Overall, therefore, the care workers in this study firmly aligned themselves with the empathic and relational skills required to do care work well rather than the more instrumental or procedural aspects embodied in the prevailing industrial-vocational approach with its national occupational standards.

At the same time, little emphasis was given to abstract or academic knowledge that would enable care work informants to apply knowledge more broadly; their responses were mostly rooted in the practical and concrete. These care workers brought values around 'helping' and 'caring' rather than theories to their work and relied on colleagues and managers for sources of inspiration. One said of watching her colleagues 'we are not all like little robots wandering around and doing everything. So I think we all put in, you know, something that you look and think, "ah yes, that's a good idea. I'll take that on board" '. No mention was made of 'training or externally gained knowledge or theories of care work as a source of inspiration or support' (Cameron and Phillips 2003: 51).

Historically, in the UK but elsewhere too, the people recruited to care work with elderly people were older women who were not in the formal labour

Table 4.2 Knowledge and skills that make you good at the job: phrases and terms used by care workers in three settings: England

Setting – type of work	Phrases and terms used
Intermediate care	Watching them. Talking to them and to relatives you tend to get a feeling for [what they can do], those that are really capable of doing it and those that just don't want to do it. Communication skills, and checking action has been carried out. Being aware of needs. Empathy, although I don't suffer from Parkinson's I understand the meaning of pain. Training in order to understand changes or symptoms.
Residential care	Good listener. Like people, like the job, get on with everybody. Talk to people as an individual, the way you'd speak to your own family, friends. Common sense, good intuition, humanity. Responsibility and understanding. It's sometimes about things that you need to be a good member of a family. Patience, listening . . . You've got to get them to trust you and once you've got that basically I think you can do anything with the resident once they trust you. Caring, understanding, patience with the residents. Speak to everybody the same, motivate them, keep them happy. Be a 'happyish go lucky' sort of person' and not 'a bit upset all the time' Social skills, empathy. Patience, timing, 'you can't rush in and get things done. I treat people how I would like to be treated'.
Home care	Listen. I am an understanding person. I listen to what they have got to say and go from there. Patience. Listening. Making a special effort to brighten what has been a miserable day for them. Formal education, health science, first aid, handling and so on. Experience with own parents, empathy

Source: Cameron and Phillips 2003

market, often 'housewives', who had developed a competence through caring in families and who were prepared to work for low levels of pay. As a Swedish civil servant put it in 1951, these 'middle aged and older housewives' should be 'able to take some hours off and . . . be content with relatively modest remuneration . . . but . . . [be] interested in the task and . . . derive benefit from the relatively modest income' (Hjalmar Mehr, cited in Johansson and Moss 2004). This group is still a primary source of recruits for care work with older people in England. If their practice wisdom from experience of familial care work is seen to be 'the same' as that required for paid work with elderly people, it can therefore be assumed that tacit knowledge is appropriate and limited further education was needed.

Cameron and Philip's research indicated that recent changes in the work to provide a more health and personal care oriented service have not substantially altered care practitioners' perceptions of what skills and knowledge are needed: most emphasis is put on relational skills. Godfrey's (2000) study of residents' views of care workers' skills supports this finding. It concluded that training should focus on maximising relational skills as residents most appreciate practical tasks carried out while maintaining their dignity and respect, and with sensitive attention to communication.

Whether tacit knowledge can continue to be viewed as an adequate basis for elder care work is questioned by the introduction of qualifications into regulatory standards (albeit at a low level and for only part of the overall workforce) and by other developments. In particular, work in this sector is getting more difficult. Policy developments such as the National Service Framework (Department of Health 2001a) which promotes independence, an individual approach to care and an increased emphasis on merging what was previously seen as 'health' with 'care' tasks, and demographic trends including increased longevity, mean that many older people living in their own homes and in residential care have higher levels of 'need' than previously. Care workers are increasingly presented with clients with medical conditions (such as dementia) that may require specialist knowledge in order to help them with daily lives. Moreover, paid work in domestic settings with older people draws workers into relationships and environments that may be difficult to manage without professional boundaries; this argument is also familiar among English childminders (Mooney et al. 2001) and among foster carers (see chapter 8).

As care work becomes more specialised and demanding, it is possible that reliance on tacit knowledge declines. A study of the use of tacit knowledge by social workers showed that they 'call upon a rich repertoire of interventions' (Zeira and Rosen 2000: 119) and that practice wisdom, often described as haphazard, or leading to undifferentiated choices of intervention, was less in evidence than rationally selected interventions. According to Carew (1979), qualified social workers use experiential knowledge and advice from more experienced colleagues to validate and apply theoretical knowledge. As Johansson (2002) argued, both formal and tacit knowledge are important, and the care worker may draw on both to differing degrees depending on the context.

At the same time, trends in general educational qualifications and labour market participation among women mean that there are fewer women with 'housewifely' experience on which to draw as a pool of labour (Coomans 2002). In countries where more formal education is required as preparation for care work, such as Sweden, there is some concern about the 'academisation' of care work. Concerns have also been expressed that the upgrading of formal education bringing improved status for workers may also risk downgrading the relational and creative side, expressing perhaps more feminine values of care work, in favour of more masculine values such as science and theorising (Wærness 1984). Wærness (1995) has also argued that a longer education for care work does not create a stable workforce as it encourages graduates to work in administration rather than practice; as we have already seen, the process of enhancing education led to a workforce haemorrhage in residential child care in England in the 1980s and 1990s.

Whether the skills and knowledge necessary are imbued through practice wisdom or are learned through formal education depends to a large extent on the value placed on the work, its constituent elements and on education overall. Wærness (1980) has argued that where care work is seen as 'work without any result', for example in the case of work with older people, it is not valued highly in society and that includes attention paid to formal education for the work. One might, therefore, expect education to focus on the workplace and essential practical tasks, rather than wider issues such as professional communication skills. However, these latter skills are likely to be increasingly important in order to achieve policy goals of choice and independence for older people.

Pedagogic work with young children in Denmark

Sitting at the professional education end of the knowledge continuum is the education to become a Danish pedagogue. The pedagogue, and the discipline of pedagogy, are discussed at length in chapter 6, in particular in relation to residential child care work in continental Europe. In Denmark, where the profession is most extensive and highly developed, the pedagogue has a three and a half year initial education leading to a degree-level qualification for work in many settings providing for people across the life course, including young children in childcare centres, but also older children, adolescents, young people and adults in both day and residential institutions. In childcare centres, pedagogues make up around half the workforce, the remainder being pedagogue assistants with no specialist education or an upper secondary level qualification. Indeed, rather than care work, the view in Denmark would be that the workforce in these centres are engaged in pedagogical work.

The initial education for pedagogues, offered in specialist colleges (*pædagog-seminarium*), combines academic studies, professional skills and practical training, and aims to integrate theory, practice and personal qualities. Great importance is attached to the development of the ability to reflect so that the pedagogue can apply theory, practice and personal qualities to particular situations and relationships. Most students begin this degree-level training when in their mid twenties; most therefore will have acquired considerable life experience, including employment, and quite a number have previously worked as pedagogue assistants. These students are thus at a very different life course position than most elder care workers in the UK (who often enter the work in their 30s and 40s) or indeed most childcare workers (who often go into the work after leaving school at 16 or 18).

The second case study from Care Work in Europe drawn upon for this chapter (Jensen and Hansen 2003) had a similar set of informants as that with older people discussed above, and included a detailed examination of pedagogues' views about the knowledge and skills important for their work. They identified nine areas of knowledge and skills that encompass academic, professional, creative and personal skills. Table 4.3 sets out some of the details given under each of these types of knowledge.

The knowledge base for working with young children as presented in this table is multifaceted and complex. Skills include many that were mentioned in relation to work with older people in England, such as listening and

Table 4.3 Knowledge and skills that make you good at the job by areas of knowledge: phrases and terms used by qualified pedagogues working in nurseries: Denmark

Areas of knowledge	Phrases and terms used by pedagogues to explain skills and knowledge needed for work with young children
Life and work experience	Background in farming; parents doing care work or teaching; caring for siblings; training as a relaxation therapist; training as a hairdresser. All experience said to be useful familiarisation, introduce a holistic view and principles of personal attentiveness.
Personality, involvement and professional identity	Empathy, personal engagement, enthusiasm, listening, show consideration and respect for children, 'must be able to offer and give something of yourself'. Keep some professional boundaries: 'need to keep things apart', 'be conscientious about what we do when we are together with the children'. Should 'radiate security', take children seriously, 'if I take the time to stop and consider the children, then I am faced with an incredible ability to co-operate and willingness to assist me'.
Reflexivity and comprehensive view	Listen to colleagues' views, be attentive, learn from them, stand firm when believe something is wrong. Keep up to date with public and local debates. Have an overview of what each person is doing, where they are and who is responsible for what during each day. Attend to specific tasks and retain some responsibility for the overall picture. Be sensitive to colleagues' interests and initiatives.
Social and expressive competences	Empathy, take child's perspective, talk with children, not decide everything, curiosity, be outgoing, patient, create a peaceful atmosphere.
Professional communication	Emphasised in education reforms of 1992. Constantly learning how to communicate effectively and accurately. Communication necessary in daily spontaneous contact, in formal discussions, in general talks to parents, and talks about specific problems. 'How to put things to parents in a sensible way so that you get dialogue and not just resistance'.

Observation and description	Describe findings, experience, and interpretations. Increasing interest in anthropologically based observations rather than child development. 'Try and see things from the child's perspective'. 'Sit down with children and pretend you are a stranger . . . to try and observe everything, to record everything, to wonder and ask . . . wonder loudly while interpreting afterwards . . . not to be too sure in your interpretations'.
Negotiation and collaboration	There are no certain objective answers, cannot follow strict plans in pedagogic institutions. Democratic tradition means lots of discussions, values and actions continually up for discussion. Self-government; 'everybody demands influence and wants influence'. Decisions are 'jointly taken and continuously modified'. Colleagues seen as clever and source of inspiration, collaboration necessary.
Professional knowledge	This was little remarked upon and possibly seen as an 'obvious' competence. 'You do need a fundamental knowledge of childhood development, because it is your responsibility together with the parents to ensure that the child thrives and evolves normally. You need to possess some kind of basic knowledge. [. . .] I also believe that you need to stick to some of the old theories which are still valid in many ways, although much that is new has also been added'.
General knowledge, practical and artistic skills and creativity	Many kinds of practical and creative skills are employed in the projects children do: e.g., drama, singing, dancing, woodwork, using the outdoors, building fires, examining plants. Pedagogues have to continually educate themselves to keep up with children's interests as well as developing particular areas of expertise for themselves (e.g, music, drama). The pedagogue 'acts as a guide and source of inspiration' for children.

Source: Jensen and Hensen 2003

observing, being attentive and responsive, communicating well and being empathetic. Pedagogues must also negotiate with colleagues, children and parents. Where the pedagogue diverges from the English care worker is that the former has also to be highly skilled in collaborative working, in being flexible and in reflexivity: she or he must be able to think critically about their work and their relationship to it, and be able and willing to engage in almost constant discussion (Korintus and Moss 2003).

In addition to the skills listed, pedagogues described many academic and professional sources of inspiration:

colleagues, children and students, from the daily working life, at staff meetings and staff weekends . . . professional magazines and professional books and follow the public debates. They participate in seminars, lectures and theme evenings. Experts on various subjects are invited to speak. They visit other institutions and in turn are visited. . . . study tours both at home and abroad. They participate in the projects initiated by municipalities.

(Korintus and Moss 2003: 78–79)

Pedagogical work in Denmark relies on combining abstract principles, and understandings of normative developments in children and childhood, with a contingent approach to understanding the dynamics of social relationships and institutions. The democratic and self-governing traditions in these institutions, and the absence of a formally prescribed curriculum, creates a requirement for pedagogues to be articulate and self-confident, highly socially aware and able to challenge as well as listen, observe and interpret as well as describe children, acknowledge difficulties in areas such as communication with parents, and try new methods where appropriate – and to reflect on and discuss their working practice. Being reflexive involves practising the art of puzzling, both internally and externally, before reaching a decision; it occupies an intellectual space before decision or judgement.

The freedom that comes from not planning details in advance also brings responsibilities to work as a close-knit team, and for each pedagogue to be aware of who is doing what and where they are, taking into account each person's skills and interests. Pedagogues must also have a personality that is attractive to children, and which 'radiates security'. Different attributes and skills should be represented in the team, as this pedagogue explains:

> I can be a bit crazy every now and then, but I also have a profound inner peace which I can apply in the work I do. Other people possess a lot of extrovert energy, which they utilize in their work. In those cases, we can complement each other if we are properly teamed up.

The pedagogues contributing to this study (Care Work in Europe) convey a conceptualisation of childhood where children are active participants in the construction of their social world, where there is respect for values, individuality and uncertainty and as a consequence everything must be debated with children as well as with adults.

Underpinning the knowledge required to be a pedagogue is an understanding of the child and her or his relation to society, and to the adults they come into daily contact with in children's services. Adults and children are increasingly seen as co-constructing their relationships and environment, and children are seen as entitled to the 'good life': a life which values living in the outdoors, being strong minded and characterful, and one where individuality is appreciated (Jensen, p.c). In Wærness' terms, and unlike work with older people, work with children is 'care work with a result', in that children are developing and progressing in a tangible way. As such it is more highly valued and education is given a more theoretical orientation, with substantial contributions from pedagogy, sociology and psychology to understand the child in relation to family, society and in relation to normative development.

Some comparative comments

Danish pedagogues participating in the Care Work in Europe study produced a much fuller list of knowledge and skill requirements than in the parallel study of care assistants in England. In part, this greater articulation may itself be an effect of their longer education, which focused on developing analytic and reflexive skills. This may mean they are better at expressing themselves in a research interview situation. Differences in responses may also be attributable to variations in life course positions, in general educational background and so on.

However, it is still the case that a much broader and deeper knowledge base is called upon to be a Danish pedagogue than an English care worker. In the Danish case, the knowledge required was more heavily weighted towards theoretical knowledge and theorising the interpersonal and less towards the discrete information end of Greenwood's continuum. In the English example, most attention was focused on practical and interpersonal skills rather than abstract knowledge, with some identification of information needs in order to be aware of changes in symptoms. Sources of inspiration and new ideas were highly localised, while for pedagogues inspiration could come from many quarters, local, national and even international.

Also significant is the relative attention paid to continuous professional development after initial education. Danish pedagogues, in whatever setting they work, have access to a wide range of higher education including postgraduate diplomas and degrees. English care workers had nearly all had access to ongoing training, and nearly all were satisfied with it. But training whilst in post was designed for entrants with very limited educational preparation for the work, was of short duration (one or two days), and was aimed at the instrumental needs of the service (such as health and safety), at extending knowledge of specific conditions and much less about general skills in how work with older people (Cameron and Phillips 2003).

Conclusions

This chapter has considered knowledge for care work on a continuum from, broadly speaking, theoretical to prescriptive. Using cross-national evidence, it has compared the case of education for work with young children at the professional-theoretical end, with the case of education, more usually referred to as training, for work with older people at the more vocational-industrial-technical-prescriptive end. The advantage of using a continuum model is to enable a cross-sectoral analysis of skills and knowledge which shows that, despite the historic fragmentation of care work, there is much in common between care workers' skills across the life course. Where the pedagogue in Denmark shows a clear departure from the care worker in England is the pedagogue's exposure to many different ways of thinking about and debating practice, while the care worker with older people picks up new ideas from the immediate working environment largely on her own initiative. The historic legacy of practice wisdom for defining care work skills is still very much in evidence in England, particularly in work with older people.

In concluding this chapter it is important to ask: why, in the UK, is there such a large gulf in the education and training for work with young children on the one hand and older people on the other? Moreover, the gap appears to be widening, with Level 3 qualifications increasingly becoming the minimum level for work with young children, and Level 5 qualifications (including degrees) extending. By contrast, work with older people is subject to severe economic and policy pressures, which may make achieving regulatory standards for education and training very difficult, or obviate the need for them altogether. For example, with the introduction of 'cash for care' or direct payments, older people control the care service they receive, and so requirements for qualifications and training are determined by the cared-for person. There is no obligation or incentive for such care workers, who may, in future, not be called 'care' workers at all, to be educated and qualified for their work.

Deciding what knowledge and education is needed to be a care worker depends on many factors outside the field of care work. Of particular importance is the societal value placed on those who are worked with – in our cases young children and older people – and societal understandings of the work and the worker. Work that is less valued and which is understood as essentially experiential or involving the application of basic procedures usually gets lower levels of education, which usually translates into low paid and low status work.

Note

1   Throughout this volume, childcare (one word) is used to denote non-school-based early education and care services, and child care (two words) refers to child welfare (social care) services for 'children in need'.

5 Location, location, location

The importance of place in care work with children

June Statham and Ann Mooney

Introduction

Caring demands a setting, 'a physical space to embody caring tasks' (Peace 1998: 107). In the case of informal care, this is most often a domestic setting, either the care provider's or the care recipient's own home. In the case of formal care services, the situation is more varied and complex. The issue of where care work takes place is fundamental to the policy of community care, which prioritises community-based domestic settings over institutional care for a wide variety of groups including older people, those who are disabled and those who are mentally ill.

The significance of location has been less explicitly acknowledged in debates about care, education and welfare services for children. However, the notion of place is becoming increasingly central to many current policy issues concerning children's needs and services. For example, is it preferable to expand nursery provision based in institutions such as schools or children's centres or increase parental leave and allowances, which would promote home-based care for very young children? How can disabled children be included in mainstream rather than specialist settings? Are residential children's homes able to provide a suitable alternative for children who need to be looked after by the state? Should different care, education and welfare services for young children be provided in one place – such as an integrated children's centre – or in separate settings? The development of Extended Schools in England, providing a base for a range of services such as childcare, parent education and family support as well as children's education, is the most recent reflection of the growing attention being given to location in public policy in developing care and other services for children.

The location of care work is important for a number of reasons. It reflects particular understandings of the nature of children's needs, whether this is for 'substitute' mothering or a complex web of relationships with other people. It has implications for a range of current policy issues, including recruitment and retention of the care workforce, the move towards increasing professionalisation of care work, and helping workers to manage their work and family responsibilities. A consideration of where care work takes place is particularly timely given the shifting and increasingly fluid boundaries between different forms of care and education services for children.

This chapter explores the location of care work with children, drawing on a wide range of recently completed and ongoing research. This includes studies of childminding, playgroups, nursery and out-of-school childcare services; family support services such as sponsored childminding, short-break foster care and mentoring projects; and studies of residential care including a cross-cultural comparison of ways of working in children's homes in Europe and a historical study interviewing former residents of the Thomas Coram Foundling Hospital in London. The chapter considers family (home-based) and institutional (group-based) care in two fields. The first is the care of children while their parents are working – often referred to as 'childcare'. Such care is usually paid for by parents. The second is care provided for children who are 'in need' or 'looked after' – often referred to as child care, and usually funded by the state[1]. In England, these two sets of services tend to be viewed as conceptually distinct, despite the fact that they are both now within the remit of the same government department, the Department for Education and Skills (DfES).[2]

The location of *responsibility* for children's services, at both central and local government level, is an important issue with implications for how the work is understood and for the pay and conditions of workers. There is a trend in most European countries towards integrating 'care' and 'education' services within one department or structure, especially services for young children. The issues that this raises have been well explored elsewhere (e.g. Cohen et al. 2004). In this chapter, we are concerned with another aspect of location: the physical settings in which care services are provided. The chapter begins with a brief overview of the historical context and the different settings in which non-parental care for children has been provided in England, and of the research evidence about children's views on their care settings. This is followed by an analysis of current locations for care work with children, and an overview of other dimensions of care that interact with location. We then consider how the place where care work is undertaken both influences and is influenced by understandings of what is best for children, the status and training of childcare workers, and the extent to which the care is subject to regulation. The chapter concludes with a discussion of the blurring of boundaries between institutional and home-based care work, and the significance of the location of care work with children for current policy concerns.

Sites of care: changes over time

Childcare for working parents

In the nineteenth century, childcare throughout the UK tended to be provided in private homes with a reliance on family, friends, neighbours and childminders for the working class, and on nannies for the middle classes. The Infant Life Protection Act, introduced in 1872, addressed the problem of 'baby farming', a practice whereby women were paid to take children into their homes while their mothers worked, and in some cases to care full time for the illegitimate babies of middle-class women. Conditions were often crowded and unsanitary (Cameron 2003). With the exception of dame schools (Tizard et al. 1976), childcare was rarely provided in non-domestic settings. Public day nurseries were opened during the Second World War, but this reflected a temporary need to increase women's employment. Once the war was over, most of these nurseries were closed and mothers were expected to care for their children at home unless exceptional circumstances made this impossible (Ministry of Health 1945). This continued to be government policy through the next decades. For example, a circular from the Ministry of Health in 1968 reiterated the government's opposition to childcare, except to support lone mothers or those with medical needs: 'Wherever possible, the younger preschool child should be at home with his mother and the needs of older preschool children should be met by part-time attendance at nursery schools and classes' (Ministry of Health 1968).

The introduction of the National Childcare Strategy in 1998 heralded the beginning of substantially increased government involvement in developing childcare services, with the aim of achieving 'quality, affordable childcare for children aged 0 to 14 in every neighbourhood' (Department of Education and Employment 1998). Part-time nursery education is now available for all 3- and 4-year-olds whose parents want it, and is beginning to be developed for 2-year-olds. There has been a particular emphasis on centre-based care, reflected in initiatives to support Early Excellence Centres and Neighbourhood Nurseries and, more recently, in government plans to establish 3,500 Children's Centres in disadvantaged neighbourhoods by 2008. These will bring together childcare with early years education, family support and health services, and act as a 'service hub' within the community for parents and other providers of childcare services (Cabinet Office Strategy Unit 2002).

Care for children in need and looked after

The location of services for children who need more focused support, and in particular those who are unable to live with their parents, has developed in a somewhat different pattern to that of services caring for children while their parents work. In the nineteenth century, institutional care predominated, with homes set up by children's charities like Barnado's to 'rescue' children from poverty and give them a better life. The Foundling Hospital established in London in 1741 by Captain Thomas Coram was one of the first such institutions. It took in babies abandoned on the streets of London or those left by unmarried mothers and provided them with care and education until the age of 14 (Oliver 2003). Few of the large nineteenth century charities worked with families in their own homes: the National Society for the Prevention of Cruelty to Children (NSPCC) was unusual in doing so rather than setting up childcare institutions (Gardner 2002). In the mid-twentieth century, however, a growing awareness of the negative effects of institutionalisation led to a move away from institutions towards more individualised care and a preference for family settings. The Foundling Hospital, for example, began to phase out residential care for older as well as younger children in the few years before the Children Act 1948 (which brought voluntary childcare charities like the Foundling Hospital within a regulatory framework for the first time), and replaced it with a combination of foster care and day school, to which children from outside the care home were admitted (Oliver 2003). Elsewhere, the 'grouped cottage' system (where children lived in separate units on a large 'campus') found favour (Parker 2003). This was seen to provide more personalised family settings, although children could still remain cut off from the wider community.

Current government policy on children in need, as expressed in the Children Act 1989, is to provide support to enable them to remain within their own families wherever possible. Where children need to be looked after away from home, foster care is regarded as preferable to residential care, especially for children under the age of ten. A few local authorities have attempted to phase out residential care for children altogether, but research suggests that both types of care need to be available (Berridge 1994). There has in any case been a significant change in the nature and size of children's homes in recent decades. Most now care for small numbers of children and operate from 'ordinary' houses within the community – although the experience of children looked after in such settings may still be significantly different from care within a domestic setting, as we discuss later in this chapter.

Sites of care: children's perspectives

There is relatively little UK research that has specifically sought children's views about where they would prefer to be cared for when not being looked after by their parents. This is particularly the case for young children receiving childcare while their parents work. One study of why children thought they were attending out-of-home care and what they said they enjoyed found no difference between four different types of early childhood setting, including nursery classes and day nurseries (Dupree et al. 2001). Reviews of the literature of children's views on the quality of childcare provision found that the following features were consistently identified as important: opportunities to be with friends, having a range of interesting activities available to them, staff who are responsive to their needs, and space and facilities conducive to play and relaxation (Clarke et al. 2003; Mooney and Blackburn 2003). This suggests that whatever the setting, it is important that it is able to provide a range of social opportunities including the chance to interact with other children.

Other studies have explored the views of children and young people who are placed in foster or residential care (e.g. Edmond 2003; Sinclair et al. 2004; Smith et al. 2004). Some of these young people do not want a replacement family and prefer the peer dynamics and wider social networks of a residential setting, reinforcing the need for choice between a range of different locations (Berridge 1994). Research on short-break foster care (Aldgate and Bradley 1999) has suggested that there may sometimes be a tension between children's and parents' needs in terms of where they would prefer to be looked after. This same study found that children would often prefer to stay within their own home, even though they generally liked their part-time foster carer and could see that it gave their parents a much needed break. Overall, however, the views of children and young people about where they are cared for remain under-researched.

The current locations of care work with children

Care work with children in the UK spans a wide range of locations. Childcare, in particular, consists of a patchwork of different services provided in a variety of settings. Many parents use a combination of services to meet their childcare needs – perhaps a childminder in the early morning, followed by a half-day session in a nursery class and then a playgroup in the afternoon. It is not unusual for a child to experience several different locations within a single day. As well as the potential disruption and lack of continuity for the child, this places a heavy burden on parents to coordinate arrangements and to transport children between services, especially if they have more than one child needing care (Skinner 2003).

Table 5.1 provides examples of care services for children, both those providing childcare whilst parents work and those providing care and support to children in need, classified according to the location of the care. Their key characteristics are outlined briefly below, before considering how the

Table 5.1 Examples of differing locations for care work with children

	Care recipient's home	Care worker's home	Non-domestic care setting	Public space
Childcare for working parents	Nanny/au pair Home carer	Childminder Private fostering	Day nursery Playgroup Out-of-school club	Adventure playground
Care for vulnerable children	Family support worker Home visitor	Sponsored childminder Respite carer Foster carer	Children's home Local authority day nursery or family centre	Mentoring project

location of these services affects the experience of children and the ways in which the work is understood.

Own home care

Parents who want their child to be cared for within their own home may choose nannies or au pairs, who are not (at the time of writing) required to be registered or inspected by government agencies. Nannies and au pairs are employed by parents, who are responsible for their terms and conditions of employment. Some nannies care for the children of two families in the home of one of them, thus bridging the divide between care in the child's own or another's home. Parents may also use a registered childcare provider called a 'home carer'. This category of carer was introduced by the government in April 2003 and was seen as a way of extending eligibility for childcare tax credit to parents who wanted their child to be cared for at home, particularly those working non-standards hours or who had a disabled child. However, take-up of the scheme by childcare providers has so far been very low (Vevers 2003).

In-home services are also available to support children designated as 'in need', that is, provided or commissioned by local authorities to meet their duty under the Children Act 1989 to provide support to children whose health or development would be significantly impaired without it (Department of Health 1991b). This includes childcare services, care provided by family support workers who visit families at home to provide help with parenting and other difficulties; and home visiting schemes like Home Start, where volunteers befriend and support families with young children who are experiencing significant difficulties in their lives (Frost et al. 1996).

Care in another's home

Childminders, also known as family day care providers, are registered to look after other people's children in their own homes. They offer the most popular form of non-parental care used by working parents, after informal care by relatives and friends (Woodland et al. 2002). Childminders can care for up to six children (including no more than three under fives) at any one time, and they may provide care before and after school and in the school holidays as well as during the working day for preschool children. However, numbers of registered childminders have been falling in recent years (Mooney et al. 2001), and concerns have been expressed about the viability of this form of home-based care to survive in a changing world (Moss 2003).

Services offered by local authorities to promote the welfare of children in need can also involve care in another family's home. Sponsored childminders (sometimes known as community or specialist childminders) are paid by public authorities such as social services departments to care for a child as a form of support for families at a time of crisis (Statham et al. 2001). Such care is usually offered for several half days a week, until the family is judged able to cope again without such help. Short-break or 'support' foster care offers a similar respite service, but often for older children and including overnight stays – typically, a weekend every fortnight or month with a support care family for a period of up to six months (Greenfields and Statham 2004). Both these forms of care are time-limited, and children remain the responsibility of their parents. Full-time foster care, on the other hand, aims to offer a replacement home for children whose parents are unable to care adequately for them. Full-time foster carers may have another job outside the home, but the essence of their foster care work is that they are providing 24-hour care to a child within their own home. Private fostering (see chapter 8) falls somewhere between childminding and foster care organised by the state. It is a private arrangement between parent and carer, but the child lives full time in another's home.

Care in a non-domestic setting

Centre-based care services include private day nurseries offering full-day care for children from birth to five years old, and playgroups providing mainly part-time provision for 2- to 4-year old children. The latter are usually run by non-profit organisations and are often located in premises designed for another purpose, such as village halls, where they need to clear away toys and equipment at the end of each session (Brophy et al. 1992). Care for school-aged children before and after school and in the school holidays is provided by a variety of clubs and schemes, sometimes but not always based in school premises (Petrie 1994). New forms of centre-based provision for children that offer a wide range of services are also being developed, such as Early Excellence Centres and Children's Centres.

For children in need who require support to enable them to remain living with their families, most local authorities still provide some childcare in day nurseries or family centres, which they run either themselves or in partnership with a voluntary organisation. As with the allocation of places in home-based care (sponsored childminding), local authorities are increasingly targeting such support at families with a high level of need and using other mechanisms, such as childcare tax credits, to support low-income or lone parent families who need childcare so they can work. When children are unable to live with their parents, residential childcare offers an alternative location to foster care within a family home. It is generally used for older children and those whose needs are judged to be too challenging for most foster carers to meet, as well as sibling groups who would otherwise need to be split between more than one foster family.

Care in a public space

Finally, care can also be provided for children within public settings such as parks. Adventure playgrounds are often located in such settings, and family support workers may take children out to leisure centres or libraries as a way of developing a relationship with the child as well as giving the parents a break from childcare responsibilities. Mentoring is an area of care work that is becoming an important element of government strategy for supporting vulnerable young people (Philip et al. 2004, and see chapter 7). Mentors are often 'matched' with a young person and meet up with them on a regular basis, sometimes at a mentoring project base but just as often in a public space such as a sports centre, café, library or cinema. As chapter 7 notes, location can be significant as a way of defusing the intensity of relationships between mentor and mentee. Engaging in activities together in a public place could be a means of creating a non-threatening context for the mentor to offer advice and support.

Location: cross-cutting dimensions

A number of other dimensions cut across the classification of care work by location presented in Table 5.1. One is the age of the child being cared for: as we show later, home-based childcare is generally seen as more appropriate than centre-based care for very young children, and children under the age of eight are very rarely placed in residential children's homes. Another cross-cutting dimension is the time that care is needed, both the duration and the time of day. Duration may be daily, as in childcare for working parents; intermittently, as in respite or short-break care for vulnerable children; or continuously, as in foster and residential care.

The time of day when care is required can also influence views on the most appropriate location. A study of barriers to developing childcare services to meet the needs of parents working atypical hours found that childcare providers were often reluctant to offer care in the late evening, overnight or at weekends; not only because of the potential impact on their own families, but also because there was a general feeling that children should be at home with their parents or a close relative at these times (Statham and Mooney 2003). If children did need to be cared for outside of the family at such times, the domestic setting offered by childminders was generally preferred.

A third dimension that interacts with location to influence attitudes towards care is who chooses or pays for the service, and the employment status of the care provider. The system of direct payments or 'cash for care' has enabled disabled people to take control of the money that would have been used by the local or health authority to purchase their care and personal support. According to service users, this represents a significant shift of power that introduces a different dynamic to the receipt of care services, especially those provided in the cared-for person's own home (Macfarlane 1993; Morris 1993). In the case of childcare, there may be a complex relationship between who pays for care, where it is located and how it is perceived, as illustrated by the reluctance of some parents to accept a free place for their child with a childminder paid by the local authority (see below).

A fourth dimension which cuts across location is the extent to which the care service is subject to registration and inspection. As we discuss, care provided in a child's own home appears to be the least regulated, and domestic settings are generally less regulated than institutional ones. But there is a growing trend towards increased regulation of all types of care services for children, including those provided in private domestic settings.

Having outlined the main locations of care work with children and some of the factors that interact with this, we turn now to a number of issues related to where care work takes place. This analysis draws in particular on the following TCRU studies: research on family day care, referred to as the 'Childminding in the 1990's' study (Mooney et al. 2001); a study of care purchased by local authorities for children in need, the 'Sponsored Daycare' study (Statham et al. 2001); a study of pedagogical[3] approaches to residential care in Europe, the Social Pedagogy study (Petrie et al. forthcoming) and a study interviewing former residents of one of the earliest children's homes in England, the 'Foundling Hospital' study (Oliver 2003).

Understandings of care: what do children need?

At one level, the many different locations where care work with children can take place offers diversity and choice: a variety of settings to meet different needs. But location also constructs and reflects different ways of being with and caring for children. Views about where children should be looked after when away from their families, either temporarily (while their parents work) or on a longer-term basis (if they cannot be cared for by their own family) reflect particular understandings about the needs of children and the ability of different types of care to meet these needs.

For example, there is a strong presumption, in some European countries at least, that young children are best cared for in their own homes by their mother. Singer (1992) has described the idea that mother care is needed for secure development and that, in its absence, non-maternal care needs to be based on a dyadic mother–child relationship as 'attachment pedagogy'. Such ideas have had a strong influence on views about where young children should receive their care, as shown in a number of TCRU studies of early years care and education. Mothers choose playgroups, for example, when their children are aged two or three so that they can mix with other children and begin to socialise outside the home (Brophy et al. 1992). Whilst some would prefer nursery education, others felt that school was not the best place for children at this age. One mother said: 'I prefer playgroup because the mothers join in and the children are too young to be off your hands completely' (Brophy et al. 1992: 67).

In the case of very young children, care by childminders is often parents' first choice if care by relatives is unavailable (Woodland et al. 2002). Parents in the Childminding in the 1990s study (Mooney et al. 2001) said they chose this form of care because of the individual attention it provided for their child and the home setting. Childminders as well as parents viewed the location of care as significant. Three-quarters of childminders surveyed in this study thought it 'very important' that they provided children with a 'home away from home'. Many conceptualised the care they provided as substitute mothering, describing themselves as 'second mums' and the children they cared for as 'like my own'. They were aware that there was a difference – as one said, 'it feels like having your own child, but you give him away at the end of the day and you get paid for it'. But the identification of this form of home-based care with mothering was strong.

One consequence was that parents in the Sponsored Daycare study (Statham et al. 2001) were often reluctant to accept support in the form of a place for their child in home-based care. Since sponsored places were offered not to parents who needed childcare so they could work, but to parents who needed support at a time of crisis, accepting such care could be interpreted as failing as a parent. One mother described how she 'felt I'd given up on him [her son]. I felt bad because I wasn't coping. I managed the others [her older children] without help'. Another mother said she would have preferred a nursery place because 'I felt that whatever she [childminder] could do, I could do'. A third felt that home-based care was less able than other types of care to meet children's educational needs: 'If you leave a child at home with a childminder she has activities: cooking, cleaning, ironing. She does not have time to teach the children.'

Social workers in this same study, however, strongly favoured the use of childminders when arranging a childcare placement for a child aged under two. This was partly because relatively few places were available in nurseries for this age group, but it also reflected a perception that very young children are best cared for in a one-to-one relationship in a home-based setting. As an officer responsible for organising sponsored placements in one of the local authorities explained:

> With younger children, our professional instincts are to steer towards childminders . . . I think it is a much more normal experience and meets the needs of the child for attachment to a limited number of adults.

If a child was still entitled to a sponsored placement when they reached the age of two or three, they would often be transferred to a group setting (in particular a playgroup) or moved into education services such as a nursery or reception class at school. Such policies reflect normative views of what young children need (Moss et al. 2000). The 'normal' young child is assumed to develop naturally if in the family, without the need for external experiences or relationships, and to then benefit from part-time (rather than full-time) care and education in a group setting for a couple of years before starting full-time schooling. This contrasts with the situation in other countries, for example the early childhood centres in Reggio Emilia in Italy, where group care is seen as a desirable way of introducing even very young children to the values of collectivity and inclusion (Dahlberg 2000).

The perception that family-based care is needed for young children can also be seen in views about the appropriate location for care of children who cannot live with their parents. The Foundling Hospital study interviewed former pupils of the Coram Foundling Hospital (Oliver 2003; Oliver and Aggleton 2000). The hospital took in illegitimate children as babies, and placed them with foster families in rural areas surrounding London where they remained until the age of five. As soon as the children reached school age, however, they were separated from their foster families and suffered an abrupt transition to institutional living, with little contact with the 'outside world' until they left to enter military or domestic service at the age of 14. Their experience of growing up in an institutional setting strongly influenced their identity and their sense of belonging to wider society. The transition from familial to institutional care represented a change from individual attention to a regimented routine. Although the health care and education the Coram residents received was probably superior to that of many poor children living in the community, their accounts reflected a lack of emotional warmth or sense of feeling 'special'. As one former resident explained, 'it wasn't the care we had at home [the foster home]. It was military style. It was "here is a job I've got to do, get on with it".' For this respondent, care without love was equated with duty.

The former residents of the Foundling Hospital were marked out in many ways as living in an institutional setting. On entry to the home they were given new names, identical haircuts and a uniform. Since then children's homes have become less regimented, but even as late as the 1970s, homes typically accommodated large numbers of children (50 or more), often in dormitory-style bedrooms and with communal eating arrangements. This could make it difficult to provide individual attention, with basic care routines organised to suit the institution rather than the child, and visible symbols of children's difference such as travelling in the home's minibus rather than by car or on public transport (Elliott 2003).

In the last twenty years there have been further changes in the nature of children's homes. They have become much smaller and many now have more staff than resident children (Berridge and Brodie 1997). Larger homes accommodating 13 or more children account for less than 10 per cent of all homes (Department for Education and Skills 2001a), and some are extremely small, accommodating no more than three children. This may constitute fewer children than are placed with a single foster family.

Yet children's experiences may still differ depending on the location of their care. In the early 1990s, Colton compared the practices of residential care staff and specialist foster carers who were looking after similarly challenging children. The care practice in the special foster homes was found to be significantly more child-oriented than that in the children's homes (Colton 1992). This was not accounted for simply by differences in the number of children cared for (most homes were fairly small), or even by the attitudes of staff – if anything, the staff in the children's homes were found to hold *more* child-centred attitudes. Instead, it appeared to be the setting or location that made the difference. As the study author put it, 'the actual performance of the special foster parents and residential caregivers was strongly influenced by the contrasting realities of family and residential living' (Colton 1992: 35). The children's homes were more bureaucratic, and this was reflected in the large amount of time residential caregivers were observed to spend in 'the office' engaged in administrative type duties.

Decreasing size of homes has been accompanied by a significant increase in the volume of paperwork needed for looked-after children, and in the regulations and standards that children's homes in the UK are required to meet. This suggests that residential care is likely to continue to offer a different kind of experience to care within a foster family. But is this necessarily so? The Social Pedagogy study (Petrie et al. forthcoming) explored European models of residential care, looking at the different settings in which such care took place and the training and values that underpinned the work. Whilst the number of children cared for in children's homes has been steadily falling in the UK, the opposite trend is occurring in countries like Germany, where 60 per cent of looked-after children are in residential care compared to 35 per cent in England, and the number in residential care rose by 18,000 (27 per cent) between 1990 and 1999. In Sweden too, there has been an increase in the number of children placed in residential children's homes, mostly in the private sector, and a decrease in foster placements (Sallnas et al. 2004).

German social workers interviewed in the Social Pedagogy study commented that residential care provided by professionally trained staff could have advantages over placement with an unqualified foster family, especially for children with multiple problems. In contrast to the 'last resort' view of children's homes in England (Packman and Hall 1998), residential care in some North European countries has been conceptualised as a positive alternative to care in the family, with a focus on holistic child development rather than simply child protection. Unlike the 'maintaining' role predominant in English children's homes, residential care is concerned with 'upbringing' in a much broader and more holistic sense (see chapter 6 and Petrie et al. forthcoming).

A related development is the diversification of institutional provision in countries such as Germany, Denmark, Sweden and the Netherlands, and the development of new locations for care which combine elements of both foster and residential care. These 'mini-homes' are regulated and funded by the state, but have some of the characteristics of foster care. In Germany, for example, the *Kinderhaus* is a family home where the children's carer (a social pedagogue) lives together with a group of children that she or he is paid to look after. A number of additional staff work on a rota basis to help out and provide the main carer with time off. Sweden and Denmark have both seen the rise of small institutions, frequently run by pedagogues, who care for young people in their own home as a living. They have often previously worked in a residential setting and have decided to change to home-based care in order to be able to work more intensively with young people. Those placed with them tend to have a high level of needs, as local authorities are reluctant to pay large fees for children with fewer difficulties.

Compared to the English small residential homes in the Social Pedagogy study, these European small institutions were reported to be operating more like a family, with carers living with children around the clock supported by a limited number of 'off site' staff (Wigfall, p.c). In children's homes in England, even small ones, staff worked shifts and sleep-in rotas, taking it in turn to provide care. For the children, the home was the 'private' place where they lived. But for the staff, it was the 'public' place where they worked, and this was reflected in features that would be unlikely to be found in a private family home, such as a staff office (often with locked doors) and posters about HIV/AIDS prevention (Petrie et al. forthcoming). Interestingly, a recent review of fostering and residential care in Wales (Clough et al. 2004) expressed concerns about the increasing use being made of 'single-occupancy units', often consisting of a rented house in a rural location, where one young person is cared for by a succession of mostly agency staff. This is likely to provide an alienating and bizarre experience for the individual young person, isolated from any peer group or other non-professional contact, let alone from parents and siblings.

Home-based care – is it 'proper' work?

The setting in which care work takes place does not only influence the experience of the children being cared for. Location also has an impact on how the work is perceived, the training that is deemed necessary and the extent to which it is seen as a 'proper job'. This is a particular issue in relation to home-based care work with children, for example the care provided by childminders or by foster carers.

All types of care work in the UK tend to be poorly paid and of low status, with far lower levels of qualification required than in many other European countries (Van Ewijk et al. 2002a and see chapter 4). But care work undertaken within the home is particularly poorly rewarded in terms of pay and status. It has been argued that one of the reasons for this is its close alignment with mothering, because of the merging of paid and unpaid care in a single setting. There is a lack of physical separation between private and public work spaces, and no temporal separation either: a carer might put in the family's laundry or prepare the family dinner while keeping an eye on non-resident children (Nelson 1994).

Caring for someone else's child in one's own home, as childminders and foster carers do, creates a number of tensions and dilemmas. These were illustrated by the findings of the Childminding in the 1990s study. On the one hand, the decision to work from home was often a positive choice, allowing childminders to combine care of their own children with paid work. Around two-fifths had taken up childminding because it was convenient while their own children were young. Yet the majority – nearly two-thirds – did not regard childminding as their chosen career. As one explained: 'I suppose it is a career in a way. I don't know. You don't really look at it – when you're doing it, you're just doing it. It's just something you do. I suppose it's like – you know, a mother at home, bringing up their children.' Because they were caring for children in their own home, it appeared harder for childminders to view what they did as a 'proper job'. Another said: 'I don't really treat it as work, as such, to me. It's just they're part of the family unit when they're here. And I just treat them as part of the family.'

This understanding of care work within the home as an extension of mothering had implications in terms of attitudes towards training and qualifications and the value attached to the work. Although two-thirds of childminders wanted to be viewed as professional childcare workers, the need for training and qualifications was less strongly felt, with some seeing personal experience of motherhood as the most important requirement. One new childminder said 'childminding is like – it just needs me being a mother. And I don't really know what sort of qualification you really need.'

The home base of childminders also created tensions between the affective and business aspects of the care work. Although the principle reason for childminding in the Childminding in the 1990s study was wanting to stay at home while at the same time earning an income, at the same time there was strong disapproval of a financial motivation for childminding. 'Good' childminders were described by childminders and parents alike as entering the occupation because they liked children and wanted to care for them, and not for financial reasons. This could come into conflict with the need to earn an income from the work. For example one childminder, who had felt justified in charging a reasonable rate for her services, described how she began to have doubts when she became attached to the child. 'When I got him . . . he's so nice, I started feeling guilty.' Others found it difficult to negotiate fee increases, charge for extra services or impose overtime rates. Unlike childcare workers in a centre-based service, these transactions occurred in the childminder's own home and were not mediated by an institutional context where there would normally be a management structure to deal with any problems. The conflation of 'love' and 'care', which is heightened by the domestic setting, is similarly reflected in the reluctance of private foster carers to regard their care work as a source of income (see chapter 8).

In the case of childminders caring for children placed with them by social workers, a third party is involved in the negotiations, and it is the local authority rather than the parent who pays for the care (Statham 2003). But the Sponsored Daycare study found that these childminders also experienced difficulties in drawing boundaries around the work, and often provided more care than they were contracted to do. 'I delouse and bath children. I take parents to the welfare rights office. I provide secondhand clothing and furniture. I provide coffee and chat and other things, but social workers have never expected it.' As with childminders caring for children while their parents worked, the boundaries between childminder and mother; and between home, family and clients, can be difficult to determine and maintain.

One obvious question is whether the low status and poor pay of home-based care work is an inevitable consequence of its location. We would suggest not. In the European examples of home-based care for looked-after children described above, the workers were clear that caring for children in their own home was a 'proper job'. The conditions in which the work was carried out (good support, three-year qualification as a social pedagogue, reasonable pay) both reflected and reinforced this. Among childminders, there are also possibilities for developing a more professional pedagogical approach, where home-based care of children is viewed neither as 'substitute mothering', nor as an inferior version of group care in a centre-based setting. This would involve childminders engaging in reflective practice, and working together in more collaborative relationships (for example through childminding networks) in order to determine what is distinctive about the kind of care they provide. This is beginning to happen in a number of countries, perhaps most strongly in New Zealand where family day care has been brought within a comprehensive system of public funding (Everiss and Dalli 2003).

Location and regulation

The extent to which a care service is regulated is at least in part related to its location. Several other factors besides location also come into play: the amount of care provided is one such factor. Childminders or playgroups that care for children for less than two hours a day are exempt from the need to be registered. Providers of short-break foster care, where children can be accommodated for no more than 28 consecutive days, may be expected to meet different standards by some local authorities (for example, in terms of medical fitness or number of spare bedrooms) than those providing care on a longer-term basis (Greenfields and Statham 2004). The child's age is another factor affecting regulation: childcare for children aged eight or over, for example, does not have to be registered and inspected, and higher adult/child ratios apply for the care of children under the age of two. It also matters whether the care is undertaken for financial reward or not. Childminders are not subject to regulation if they are caring for children to whom they are related, or are providing unpaid care for friends.

But alongside these factors, location exerts its own influence. Different settings for care work with children are subject to different regulatory requirements. Generally, care provided in the child's own home is the least regulated, reflecting a predominant ideology of not interfering in 'private' lives and the notion of privacy and rights within one's own home. The government can offer advice, for example on food hygiene or fire safety (and, increasingly, on parenting), but the home when used as a place of informal care for family members is not a regulated setting. This includes paid care provided for a child in their own home by a nanny or au pair, although at the time of writing the government was consulting on the development of a system of 'approval' of unregulated settings which would allow parents using these forms of care to access the childcare element of the Working Tax Credit (Sure Start 2004).

Childcare provided in another person's home has become increasingly subject to regulation, from the Infant Life Protection Act 1872 onwards. Childminders are now expected to meet national minimum standards and are subject to annual inspections by Ofsted. There are still some interesting anomalies, however, that indicate an ambivalence about the status of care provided in a domestic setting and the extent to which the government can – or should – set standards. In 2000, the DfEE consulted parents and child-minders about whether or not childminders should be allowed to smack children in their care or smoke in their presence within their own homes – practices that were not permitted within group care settings. The National Childminding Association (NCMA) itself wanted a ban on smoking and smacking, but the government decided to leave the choice with parents. At the time, the Minister for Employment and Equal Opportunities justified treating childminders differently from other childcare workers on the basis that 'childminding is a more informal setting [and] the government shouldn't have to regulate on what people can and can't do in their own homes' (DfEE press release, 14 September 2000).

Childminders were also originally excluded from eligibility to receive the nursery grant, through which the government funds providers in both the maintained and independent sectors to offer half-day educational sessions for 3- and 4-year olds. One reason for this exclusion was concerns about ensuring the educational quality of care provided in individual domestic settings. After representations from the NCMA, this decision was reversed and childminders became eligible to receive the grant, but only if they were members of an approved childminding network. Those who chose to operate as home-based providers outside such support structures remained ineligible.

Turning to the care of children who are unable to live with their parents, a similar pattern can be seen of increasing regulation being applied to domestic as well as to group settings. National Minimum Standards for Foster Care were introduced in 2002 (Department of Health 2002b). Small privately run children's homes accommodating fewer than four young people, which used to be exempt from the need to register, were brought within a regulatory framework in the Care Standards Act (2000) and are subject to the National Minimum Standards for Children's Homes (2002).

One consequence of this growing institutionalisation of domestic settings and family homes, with requirements for the installation of safety glass, fire doors and alarms and so on, is an apparent blurring of the boundaries between care work carried out in different locations. This trend might be seen as a developing in quite a different direction to that of the small institutions in Denmark, for example, where the emphasis is on de-institutionalisation in domestic settings.

New locations for care work

This blurring of boundaries between work in institutional and domestic settings is being reinforced by structural changes to the delivery of children's services in England following the government Green Paper *Every Child Matters* (Department for Education and Skills 2003) and the Children Act 2004. New ways of delivering services to children are being developed that have the potential to lead to new forms of care. Childminders are increasingly working together in more collaborative relationships, for example through childminding networks (Owen 2003), and may have links to centre-based services such as Children's Centres which mean they are no longer solely home based. Such connections are already well established in other countries such as Sweden, where family day care providers meet regularly to support each other and discuss their practice (Karllson 2003), and in Hungary, where family day care providers have strong links with the public nurseries where many of them were previously employed (Korintus 2003). In the case of foster carers, new types of care are emerging such as treatment foster care and foster carers attached to residential children's homes, especially for the most challenging young people who have previously been regarded as too difficult to care for within a family home.

Another important development in terms of the location of services is the extended role envisaged for schools, as sites for all kinds of work with children and their families. All schools are being encouraged to act as a hub for a wide range of services for children, families and other members of the community, including childcare, adult learning, health and community facilities; and the government plans to have at least one 'full service' extended school in every Local Education Authority in England by 2006 (Department for Education and Skills 2003). Similar developments have been occurring in Scotland since 1997, through the New Community Schools programme. It is argued that this extended role for schools will lead to integration of education, health and social care services around the needs of children (Department for Education and Skills 2003: 29). But concerns have also been raised, for example that it might lead to an increasing 'schoolification' of children's lives (Cohen et al. 2004), or to distortion of the goals of early childhood provision through closer contact with a formal education agenda (Organisation for Economic Co-operation and Development 2001).

The Extended Schools policies will undoubtedly lead to additional services being provided on school sites, and may reduce some of the barriers hindering children and parents from accessing family support and other services that are usually located on physically separate sites. But the proposals may not achieve a more integrated way of working with children and families unless there are also parallel changes in the cultures and training of different professions. Whilst co-location of services may be a good precursor to new ways of working with children, by itself it is no guarantee that this will happen. The physical setting of services is important, but this needs to be accompanied by reflection on what kind of experience is being sought for children. For this reason, some have argued that the term 'children's services' should be replaced with the concept of 'children's spaces', with the latter concept implying not just a physical space 'but also a social space, a cultural space and a discursive space' (Moss and Petrie 2002).

Conclusions

In this chapter, we have explored how location can produce particular ways of working and understandings of care work. We have argued that the home base of family day carers is a significant factor in why they take up the work, and in their beliefs about the kind of care they can offer to children. Similarly, the domestic nature of family life is seen by foster carers as an essential element of the care they provide for looked-after children. But the home location of such care also has particular consequences for pay, status and training.

Over time, the preferred location for the care of children has shifted, reflecting economic and political priorities as well as understandings of the needs of children. Different trajectories can be seen for the care of children while parents work and the care of children in need. The former has moved from predominantly home and family based care towards favouring group or centre-based settings, such as developing childcare in schools and through children's centres (although there is still some ambivalence about out-of-home care for very young children). Home-based formal care (childminding) has been declining. The preferred location of care for children who are unable to live with their families has moved in the opposite direction, from an institutional to a home base. But equally important is the growing erosion of boundaries between institutional and home-based care, which offers new challenges and possibilities for care work with children.

Location is an important aspect of care work. It influences and is influenced by beliefs about what is best for children, and it affects how the work is understood and the status and training of the workers. But these links often remain implicit. The connections between where care work takes place and the nature of the care experience need to be made explicit and questioned: for example, the assumption that the needs of very young children are best met by care in their own (or another's) home, rather than by a particular kind of attentive responsiveness that could be achieved in a variety of settings, given a good enough adult/child ratio and appropriate conditions. Or the assumption that foster care within a family is almost always preferable to care in a residential children's home, regardless of how the care is organised and the values that underpin it. European comparisons are often instructive in revealing the ideologies underpinning care work with children. Ziehe (1998) argues that by attempting to mirror the intimacy and 'cosiness' of the domestic home, early childhood institutions risk creating a 'false closeness', and also miss the chance to open up many new opportunities for young children 'through a complex and dense web of relationships ... within a vision of the rich child and a co-constructing pedagogy' (Dahlberg et al. 1999: 82).

This chapter has only begun to touch upon some of the issues arising from the location of care work, using examples from a range of TCRU studies of services for children. But even this initial analysis suggests that location interacts in complex ways with other aspects of care work, including who does the work, the training and qualifications required and the extent to which the setting is subject to regulation. It suggests that more critical attention could usefully be paid to the issue of where care work takes place, and to the implications of location for current policy issues. The views of children about how and where they prefer to be cared for would also repay further investigation.

Notes

1 Throughout this volume, childcare (one word) is used to denote non-school-based early education and care services, and child care (two words) refers to child welfare (social care) services for 'Children in need'.
2 Responsibility for childcare services was transferred from the Department of Health to the DfES in 1998, and for child welfare (social care) services in 2003.
3 Pedagogy refers to a holistic approach to working with children that regards learning, care and daily upbringing as inseparable (Petrie 2003).

Part II

6 The professional care worker

The social pedagogue in northern Europe

Janet Boddy, Claire Cameron and Pat Petrie

Mette is 51 years old. Married, with two teenaged children, she lives in a small town in northern Denmark. She has a degree-level diploma in social pedagogy, and has worked in residential establishments since she graduated at the age of 26. She lives a short drive from the residential institution where she worked as a 'group pedagogue' for the last nine years. More recently, she has become 'team leader' for a staff group of six pedagogues. Between them, they care for a 'living group' of eight young people, aged between five and 14 years; the institution has three living groups and a small school for residents, all on the same site. Mette works 37 hours a week, covering day and evening shifts; she no longer works overnight or at weekends. She always works with the same group of staff and young people, although pedagogues and young people in different living groups all meet regularly, and in her role of team leader she has regular meetings with other team leaders and the head of the institution. As team leader, Mette spoke of her pedagogical responsibilities for the staff group *and* for the young people. She felt the pedagogic education had been very important, for her and her colleagues, in 'using myself as a person and my professional knowledge and skills, that I give something, that I make a difference'. Mette valued her institution's emphasis on education and development, saying 'we try to keep up, to improve and become more competent. It means every day is different.' Part of her work involves supervising pedagogy students on placement in the institution, and she observed that they have to learn that 'to like the children is not enough'. During her time working in the institution, Mette had taken a number of additional training courses, ranging from a 'fabulous' one year University course in organisational pedagogy, to a football coaching certificate. After 25 years of work in residential care, Mette commented that she will probably move on to work as a training consultant in a few years time, 'before I end up as an old person here'.[1]

In chapter 4, we discussed the notion of there being a continuum of knowledge and education among care workers, and offered the example of the pedagogue as a worker in services for young children, who has received a theory and practice based professional education. Elsewhere, Moss and Petrie (2002) proposed that a pedagogic approach to work with children in general would enable the worker to move 'from technician to reflective practitioner, researcher, co-constructor of knowledge, culture and identity' (137). In this chapter, we draw on the findings of two recent studies of the social pedagogue, 'Social Pedagogy 1' and 'Social Pedagogy 2' (Petrie et al. forthcoming), working with young people looked after in residential settings, to look in more detail at this example of professional care work. The research we describe here was focused on the opportunities that may be afforded by a pedagogic approach to residential care for children and young people, but this is just one example of the work in which pedagogues are engaged. We will argue that the professionality of the pedagogue may have wider benefits for employers and employees, for example, with regard to workforce issues, such as staff turnover. Looking from the employees' perspective, we will also consider what pedagogy brings to the practice of care work, for example in terms of practitioner skills and job satisfaction.

The first part of our research on social pedagogy (Social Pedagogy 1) entailed visits to five European countries: Belgium (Flanders), Denmark, France, Germany and the Netherlands. In each country, interviews were conducted with civil servants (to learn about local and national policy), staff and students in pedagogic training and educational establishments, and managers and pedagogues working in children's residential settings. The second part of the research (Social Pedagogy 2) comprised a more formal comparison, with a mixed quantitative and qualitative design, of work in residential settings in England, Denmark and Germany, through interviews with managers, young people, and residential care workers.

What is social pedagogy?

Pedagogy is a concept that holds little currency in care work in the United Kingdom today; the term is used primarily in the context of the classroom, often referring to the science of teaching and learning in formal education (Mortimore 1999). In much of the rest of Europe, however, pedagogy has a different meaning: it relates to the overall support for children's development, and can be understood as 'education-in-its-broadest-sense'. As such, pedagogy is about 'upbringing' (*Erziehung* in Germany, the birthplace of pedagogy in the nineteenth century). A Dutch academic interviewed as part of our research described pedagogic theory as 'specially about relationships, child rearing relationships'. The home is often cited as the first site for pedagogy, and parenting (or bringing up children) is seen as pedagogic: in Germany, texts on parenting can be found in the pedagogy sections of book-shops, and the term used for German residential care workers – *Erzieher* – can be translated as 'upbringer'.

The term '*social* pedagogy' (*Sozialpedagogik* in German) is sometimes used to denote work with more vulnerable groups in society, such as children who are looked after, but different countries use different terms and have different emphases. In French, for example, the term '*éducation*' denotes pedagogy (not what the English-language world understands by the English word 'education'), while '*éducation specialisée*' is close to social pedagogy. Or, to take another example, the Flemish-speaking parts of Europe (Flanders, the Netherlands) distinguish between a number of special-isations within pedagogy, using 'social pedagogy' to refer to the 'socialising' of young people, and 'orthopedagogy' to refer to pedagogic work in three service sectors: disabilities, addictions, and 'special youth care' (which includes work with children looked after in residential settings). In recent years in Denmark, previously separate strands of pedagogic training have been unified into a generalist education taken by all pedagogues, but there remain separate trade unions for pedagogues who work in mainstream settings, such as nurseries and out-of-school facilities and social pedagogues whose professional domain is akin to social care in the UK.[2]

These cross-national variations in terminology belie a common under-standing. In many European countries, social pedagogy operates as a unifying concept that underpins theory, policy, education, and practice with children and young people with diverse levels of need and in diverse settings, includ-ing schools, childcare settings, residential care, youth work, and leisure ser-vices. In our interviews across Europe, with policy-makers, practitioners, and tutors and students of social pedagogy, certain key principles of social pedagogic practice emerged.

- A focus on the child as a whole person, and support for the child's overall development.
- The practitioner seeing herself/himself as a person, in relationship with the child/young person.
- While together, the child and practitioner are seen as inhabiting the same life space, not existing in separate hierarchical domains.
- As professionals, social pedagogues should constantly reflect on their practice, applying both theoretical understandings and self-knowledge to their work, and the challenges it poses.
- Social pedagogues are practical, and are trained to share in children's daily lives, for example, preparing meals, making music, building kites.
- When working in group settings, social pedagogues should foster and

make use of the group: the children's associative life is an important resource.

- Social pedagogy builds on an understanding of children's rights and respect for the child that is not limited to procedural matters or legislated requirements.
- An emphasis on team work, encompassing all those who contribute to the task of 'bringing up' children: other professionals, members of the local community, parents and other family members.

These social pedagogic principles accord with much of the rhetoric of current UK policy for children's services, as for example in the English Children Act (2004), with its emphasis on co-operation between 'persons or bodies of any nature ... [who are] engaged in activities in relation to children' (op. cit.: Part 2 Section 10), and in the English government Green Paper *Every Child Matters* (Department for Education and Skills 2003).[3]

In the UK, as elsewhere in Europe, personal attributes and experience are valued in care work. For example, Mooney and colleagues (2001) reported that the majority of childminders in their English research considered themselves to be professional childcare workers, but less than a quarter considered it very important to have a childcare qualification, and most felt that the experience of being a parent was more important than formal qualification. Within social pedagogy, the personal is valued – but mainly in its relationship to professional education and practice, with each informing the other. As we shall show in this chapter, tacit knowledge alone is not sufficient qualification for pedagogic care work. In the countries we studied in continental Europe, policy and practice in working with children derive from a highly developed and coherent professional education in social pedagogy.

Each of the five continental European countries studied has legislated for residential care workers to hold recognised social pedagogic qualifications, which are implemented through inspection, placement and registration criteria in residential settings for young people. In Denmark, for example, staff qualifications and ratios have been specified since the 1950s, and data from 1999 for state-run institutions show 95 qualified social pedagogues per 100 resident children. Similar facilities in France require a ratio of one qualified social pedagogue (*éducateur specialisée*) for every five or six young people. The head of a private non-profit establishment interviewed in France observed that, 'Everyone has got a degree. That's not luck, it's policy.' In the same vein, a German civil servant remarked that 'everyone should have it [the social pedagogy diploma] in order to have the appropriate skills. This will save us money in the end, because they will work well with the children, and maybe they can return home earlier.' So, what is being required by such policies? What does a professional social pedagogue's education entail?

Education for social pedagogy

A number of different levels of social pedagogic education and qualification are available in the countries studied, ranging from studies in the last years of secondary school to Masters-level academic qualifications that require five years of study. Most of those who go on to work professionally as social pedagogues have a degree-level professional diploma, based on up to four years of study. The approach to the education and training of social pedagogues is not identical in the countries studied, but the overall structure of the professional qualification is quite similar across countries. Courses have a broad theoretical base, drawing predominantly on behavioural and social sciences, such as philosophy, psychology, sociology, legal, political and economic studies. Students are also introduced to the skills needed for group working, including teamwork and communication skills. Creative and practical subjects – such as art, drama, sport, woodwork or gardening – form an important component of the pedagogy diploma, providing media through which the social pedagogue can relate to children. These subjects are also valued for their general therapeutic value: they can help young people to enjoy life and feel good about themselves.

Practice placements form a key part of the learning experience and an increasing proportion of the course as it progresses. For example, in the Netherlands, students spend half a day each week on placement in the first year, rising to one day a week in the second year, followed by ten months in the third year of their four-year diploma. Similarly, in France, third-year students for the diploma in *éducation specialisée* spend up to nine months on their final placement. Great store is placed on pedagogues being reflective practitioners, and students are taught to draw on both the personal and the theoretical in reflecting on their practice experiences. In Denmark, for example, students keep a diary of their practice placement, which takes place at the beginning of each academic year, to inform their more classroom-based learning over the remainder of the year.

Generally speaking, the social pedagogy diploma or degree is not specialised, and graduates go on to work in a variety of service sectors, but students can specialise to some extent through optional study modules, and through their practice placements within specific settings, such as youth work or work in residential care. In Denmark, the client group for pedagogues was described by several informants as '0 to 100 years', and students there have the opportunity to work in adult settings, including work with adults with disabilities and in elder care. The generalist approach to pedagogy in Denmark – going beyond children and young people and the social pedagogy focus on vulnerable groups – creates a much greater scope for vertical and horizontal mobility than occupation-specific forms of vocational qualification: the career of a Danish pedagogue might include work with young children in nurseries, adults with disabilities and residential youth care, and 'front-line' practice, management, trade union work and teaching peda-gogue students.

Continuous learning is also a key tenet of social pedagogic practice. Qualified social pedagogues develop their specialisation through ongoing education, as well as reflection with colleagues on their practice. In the words of one French social pedagogue interviewed, 'It is a job where every day you must ask questions about yourself and your practice, right to the end of your professional life.'

The first phase of our cross-national research led us to conclude that this generalist qualification (diploma or degree) might have a number of advantages as an approach to work in residential care, in relation to employment issues such as employee satisfaction and recruitment and retention problems, and – perhaps most importantly – in terms of the skills and knowledge base that pedagogues bring to the work itself. The remainder of this chapter will draw on the second phase of enquiry, which considered evidence of benefits for the practice of residential care work, associated with the profession of social pedagogy.

Residential care in England, Germany and Denmark

Policies around placement in residential care differ between England, Denmark and Germany, as do the numbers and relative proportion of children and young people who are looked after.[4] In England, which has a total population of around 50 million (84 per cent of the total UK population), 60,800 children were in local authority care in 2003. Just under 10 per cent of these young people (5,900) were accommodated in residential settings. By contrast, Denmark and Germany have much higher proportions in residential settings. In Denmark, which has a population of 5.4 million, just over 14,000 children and young people are in placements outside of their homes, of whom over 40 per cent (5,934 children, about the same number as for the whole of England) are accommodated in residential settings. In Germany, with a population of 82.5 million, 59 per cent of young people in care (82,000) are placed in residential homes.[5]

Differences between the countries in the proportion of young people in residential accommodation reflect variation in several aspects of policy. The majority of children in care in England are placed with foster carers (68 per cent), reflecting a policy preference for this form of placement (e.g. the Choice Protects initiative, launched in 2002). Residential care homes tend to be used when foster placements have repeatedly broken down (for example, because of behaviour such as school non-attendance), and as such are often seen as a placement of last resort.

The relative proportion of children and young people looked after who are fostered has increased in Germany and Denmark. But in both countries, residential settings are seen as a preferred option for some young people. In part, this reflects a pedagogic emphasis on individual care planning and on legislated requirements for children to be consulted and, in Denmark, for young people aged 15 or older to consent to care plans. These policies have given rise to a diversification of placement possibilities, to enable flexibility in choosing appropriate provision for the child or adolescent. In Germany, for example, the Federal Ministry for Family Affairs, Senior Citizens, Women and Youth finances pilot projects to develop and evaluate different forms of residential provision – such as 'five day settings', where children go home at the weekend. Similar policies in Denmark have, since the 1960s, led to the development of 'anti-institutions'; these small family-like establishments, with just a few (usually four to six) children, are today called 'social pedagogic residences'. Residential care is also preferred in some instances because it is seen as better able to meet pedagogic aims for the young people. In the first phase of our work, some German interviewees in local government commented that trained professional pedagogues in residential facilities were seen as better equipped to work therapeutically, and so to meet children's needs, than unqualified foster parents.

Workforce issues

Employment issues are sometimes analysed as a 'system', for example, based on the throughput of labour required for services to function. As we shall show, the social pedagogic approach to work in residential care is not confined to this approach and its concern with ensuring, for example, that sufficient numbers are present to meet required ratios. Rather, the social pedagogic emphasis on the personal focuses attention on the workers having attributes, skills and knowledge that enable them to relate to the young people in their care. In light of this emphasis on the personal, the analysis presented here incorporates the perspective of the workers, in order to illuminate the issues they perceive in the work they do. The data presented here are derived from interviews with unit managers and staff and a comparison of practice in residential settings for young people in England, Denmark and Germany.

Employee characteristics

Some characteristics of residential care workers were similar across the three countries, as can be seen in Table 6.1. Most workers interviewed in England and Germany were female, and there were no cross-country differences in staff ages. English respondents included a high number of workers from minority ethnic backgrounds, relative to Denmark and Germany and to the UK social care workforce (see chapter 2). This may reflect sampling, in that the study set out to include the experience of young people from minority ethnic groups, and so included a number of residential homes in inner-city locations.

More striking are the cross-national differences in workers' qualifications. Managers of residential establishments in England reported that 20 per cent

Table 6.1 Characteristics of residential care workers interviewed

	England	Germany	Denmark
% female	67	53	76
Mean age *(s.d.)*	38 *(9.33)*	39 *(7.98)*	37 *(8.02)*
% ethnically white	72	91	94
Highest qualification reported by residential care staff: n *(%)*			
No qualification	19 *(35)*	0	1 *(3)*
Other childcare qualification	0	1 *(2)*	0
Low-level qualification	4 *(7)*	0	0
Mid-level qualification	19 *(35)*	22 *(45)*	1 *(3)*
High level qualification	12 *(22)*	26 *(53)*	31 *(94)*

Source: Social Pedagogy 2

Notes:1. Data on employee age gender and ethnicity are based on staff interviewed: England = 52; Denmark = 38; Germany = 49. 2. Education levels based on SEDOC levels, which provide a common frame of reference for training, adopted by the European Community in 1985 (Van Ewijk et al. 2002a). Data on 'other' and 'other childcare' qualifications have been omitted from the table where respondents gave no information about the level of the qualification.

of staff had no known qualification. Of the English care workers interviewed, 57 per cent reported holding a mid-level (upper secondary) qualification such as an NVQ3 (35 per cent) or a high-level qualification (22 per cent), a higher figure than in earlier studies of the residential care workforce, which have indicated that less than 30 per cent hold relevant qualifications (Improvement and Development Agency 1999). In contrast, 94 per cent of workers interviewed in Denmark held a degree-level qualification in pedagogy; and 98 per cent of German staff held social pedagogy qualifications, divided between the mid-level qualification (a three-year further education *Fachschule* diploma) (58%) and a degree-level *Fachhochschule* diploma (45 per cent).

In line with the cross-country differences in initial education, fewer English care workers reported in-house training: 55 per cent compared with 75 per cent in Germany and 79 per cent in Denmark. English workers were more likely to have had training in the form of 'other short course': 72 per cent compared to 42 per cent in Germany and 58 per cent in Denmark. The discourse around education and training also differed between countries, which is perhaps not surprising, given that interviewees' perspectives are located in the specific learning culture of their country. For example, respondents in England tended to report training in instrumental terms, being taught to 'do things in the right way', as one said. Danish respondents spoke more often of gaining both personally and professionally from ongoing training, with one interviewee saying that 'we staff members become more competent all the time, and receive ongoing training [in order to] involve your feelings and thoughts in the work all the time' and another suggesting training gave their work 'more depth, understanding, maturity'. Respondents in Germany tended to emphasise the importance of practice and practical experience in their training, such as 'practical experience in the kindergarten with singing songs and messing about'. That said, there were also common-alities between England, Denmark and Germany in care workers' positive and negative views of training, for example in terms of the benefits of net-working – making contacts and sharing experiences – and a number of respondents in each country questioned the relevance of some topics of training (although the specific topics criticised varied across countries).

In all three countries, the personal attributes of staff were highlighted, and in England particularly, personal qualities were seen as the real source of strength for this group of care workers. This observation corresponds to points raised in chapter 4 concerning the English emphasis on life experience as a qualification for care work. In the absence of specific relevant qualifica-tions, personal attributes could be seen to provide the main resource for workers, and, in the words of one manager of an English home, to enable them to 'withstand the rigours of the job', and provide some emotional self-defence in an often 'draining' environment.

Pre-existing personal attributes were considered important in both Denmark and Germany, but a social pedagogic approach sees such qualities as important in combination with, and in order to make the best use of, the intellectual foundation and the personal formation involved in preparing for the work. This emphasis is illustrated by the comments of one Danish manager of a residential home: 'to be able to maintain this job – personally, professionally, and administratively – it is necessary to develop intuition and a sense of the situation – the most important elements in the work, plus theoretical knowledge'. Another commented on how 'personality and professionality go hand in hand'.

Positive personal attributes are an important characteristic of residential care workers, but to rely on recruits having such qualities as a substitute for relevant professional education may lead to difficulties in a demanding work environment. This was apparent in the responses of some English managers and care workers, who expressed concerns about staff quality; for example, one manager spoke of 'inexperienced ... poor quality staff ... staff with unrealistic views about the job'. While a worker in another estab-lishment remarked that 'the number of people here who really want to work with kids is disheartening, so people try to get by on a minimal amount of work'.

Staff turnover and satisfaction

Employers' ability to recruit and retain their workforce can be seen as an indication of work satisfaction among staff: if workers are dissatisfied they leave, or want to leave and search for another job, either of a similar kind or outside the field altogether. A high level of turnover in care services has often been said to be indicative of poor quality care and poor quality employment

(Cost Quality and Outcomes Study Team 1995; Whitebook et al. 1989). At the same time, recruitment and retention figures are likely to be influenced by wider factors such as the state of the local or national economy, career ambitions, which may be gendered, and local employment opportunities. In addition, problems of staff retention could reflect difficulties relating to the quality of work, as well as to the supply of potential workers: as some of our interviewees remarked, there are few benefits to keeping staff in post if their work is not good enough. Higher staff turnover has implications for children's experience of stability and continuity of relationships.

As shown in Table 6.2, managers' reported higher staff turnover in England than elsewhere, as well as more difficulties with recruitment and retention. This observation was supported by care workers' reports of their time in post. In England, staff interviewed had been employed for an average of just over three years, compared with seven years in Denmark and Germany (mean duration of employment (*s.d.*): England = 3.11 (*3.49*); Denmark = 7.31 (*6.05*); Germany = 6.85 (*7.81*)).

Managers of English institutions attributed recruitment problems to working conditions (including shift work, poor pay, and the risk of assault), to the perceived status of the work, and to bureaucratic difficulties of the application process. Almost all the English home managers agreed that the professional position of residential care work was one of low status, and many care workers shared this view. One manager of an inner-city home remarked that the 'bottom line is it's a thankless task', and in a similar vein, another commented that poor salary was not the only cause of retention problems, but that 'people feel undervalued'. One of several care workers who commented on the low status of the work observed that 'social work is perceived as a drop dead career', and highlighted the lack of encouragement for a career path. Several managers also remarked that the negative media portrayal of residential social work had adversely affected attempts at recruitment, for example, because 'knowledge is based on horror stories'.

Difficulties to be found in the working environment were also said to contribute to problems in recruitment and retention. In part, English

Table 6.2 Managers' reports of staff turnover, recruitment and retention

	England *(n = 24)*	*Germany* *(n = 17)*	*Denmark* *(n = 12)*
% of staff who have left in previous 12 months	28	18	11
% of managers reporting recruitment difficulties	88	45	0
% of managers reporting retention difficulties	48	8	0

respondents attributed this to policy changes over the years, resulting in residential provision often being seen today as an option of last resort, used for a minority of children and young people who present the greatest difficulties. For example, one described her clientèle as 'all boys [who have been] excluded [from school], all abused, all offenders, [previously involved in] domestic violence, boys [who had] left mums and [had been] attacking mums'. Respondents connected such characteristics among their client group to the risk of physical and verbal abuse towards staff by young people.

Concerns about recruitment and retention were not nearly so pronounced in Germany or Denmark. This may be attributable to local labour markets, as well as the higher salary and professional status of the work. That said, some German managers commented on the beginnings of problems with recruitment, in particular of male staff, and related this – as in England – to conditions of work such as stress, shift work, and low salaries. Some German residential home managers referred to actively creating a supportive working atmosphere as an aid to staff retention.

In Denmark, a similar emphasis on creating a positive working environment was discussed in the context of broader professional aims of a 'culture of involvement' and emphasising the importance, above all, 'to be professional and [for staff] to believe in [their] own professionality [and] cooperation'. None of the twelve Danish managers interviewed reported any recruitment or retention problems. This may be attributable to their management ethos and the social pedagogues' professional status. For example, we were told that 'pedagogues experience autonomy in their work and they have a possibility to make a difference . . . They prefer this work to other pedagogical [work] (e.g. in childcare centres) . . . they stay here because of the challenges.'

Accounts such as this are striking in their contrast to the difficulties described in English residential care: the Danish client group is defined less negatively, the staff group is defined as more skilful, resourceful, autonomous and reflective, and the job of the social pedagogue is defined as more attractive. A further difference relates to the discourse surrounding residential care. Danish and German pedagogues tended to describe their work in terms of success at helping young people, whereas English practitioners more often constructed their experience as dogged survival in the face of constant criticism and difficulty.

Practice issues

The idea, and the reality, of making a difference to young people's lives was a clear source of reward for German and Danish social pedagogues, in line with the emphasis of social pedagogic theory on the individual's potential for development. This was exemplified in the comments of one Danish social pedagogue who spoke of her satisfaction 'where I see that the children develop, their self-awareness, self-insight . . . to see that they get the hope and the glimmer back in their eyes, that they get the belief that there are possibilities for them in life'.

Being together with the young people in their 'living world' is also a key facet of the social pedagogic approach, and an important part of the education aims to give students practical and creative skills that they can use in everyday life in their work with children and young people. Both Danish and German social pedagogues spoke of the satisfaction they derived from this aspect of their work. One German worker said that 'it makes fun to do things together', and another that 'you can accompany children a long way'. In a similar vein, a Danish social pedagogue spoke of being 'together with the young people, maybe not for a long time, but that we are on their side and support them . . . I enjoy working with them, their power, the dialogue, the ping-pong.'

In line with their training, social pedagogues in Germany and Denmark often spoke about the young people they worked with as individuals with whom they had relationships, and emphasised the normal rather than the abnormal. Asked to describe the children they knew best, these respondents described personality traits such as curiosity and even, in one case, spoke of physical characteristics such as height. That is not to say that these young people were without difficulties, in their current behaviour and past experiences, nor that the social pedagogues did not acknowledge the challenges posed by their needs and behaviour. As one Danish pedagogue explained:

> You can feel very drained because of the problems of the children and of witnessing how tragic their fates are . . . to see a child very unhappy and sad and there [is] no [prospect that] that mother will have a better situation or improve. It touches you. Sometimes no matter how much you give or fill in, then you cannot fill these children up. There is still a gap/void and they crave for more. The days when you do not burst from energy you may get a feeling of fatigue.

Compared to social pedagogues in Denmark and Germany, English residential care workers and managers tended to offer more problematised descriptions of their work with young people in their care, referring to their past experiences (for example of parental maltreatment) and to current problems such as substance misuse, criminal offending, or absconding. For example, one worker, asked to describe the resident that (s)he knew best, spoke of 'a street child – street culture – very independent. Before coming here he was on the streets. He's not very academic, prefers hanging around with his friends, smoking weed.' Another, described a young woman resident, saying, 'she's got a bit better, communicating better with the young women and the staff now. . . . She's very hard to talk to. Quite often if you speak to her she ignores you. So it's an uphill struggle.'

Conceptualisations of the work

In chapter 4, we defined a professional education as that which prepares or enables the worker to apply and adapt their theoretical and conceptual knowledge to a range of situations, to think critically and make fine judgements, and to reflect on practice. This forms the basis of a distinction between the social pedagogic approach to residential care and the approach to this work in England, where practice and procedures are prescribed through NVQ-based training in Caring for Children and Young People, and documentation relating to the Care Standards Act (2000). For example, the National Minimum Standards for Children's Homes (Department of Health 2002b) emphasises procedures such as the requirement for documented and regularly reviewed risk assessment of

> the home's premises and grounds, children's known and likely activities (both permitted and illicit), the potential for bullying and abuse within or outside the home, and where applicable the impact of emergency admissions to the home for both the admitted child and the existing child group.
>
> (Standard 26.2)

In a similar vein, Standard 7.12 sets out regulations for therapeutic work with children, which seem a long way from the social pedagogic conceptualisation of the therapeutic value of everyday shared activity:

> Any specific therapeutic technique is only used with any child at the home if specified in the child's placement plan and specifically approved by the child's placing authority and, where the placing authority does not have parental responsibility, by the child's parent (or parent if the child is not placed by a local authority or voluntary organisation), and if the safe and effective use of the technique is known to be supported by evidence. It is carried out only by, or under the supervision of a member of staff or other practitioner holding a current recognised qualification in the therapy concerned, whose qualification the home has verified as valid and appropriate directly with the awarding body or relevant register. Any member of staff using such a technique is supervised in using the technique by a person outside the home and not responsible for the home, who is qualified and experienced in the therapy concerned.

The principles underlying such a prescriptive regulatory framework may be understandable, given past problems in residential care services. But although these regulations set out to 'enable rather than prevent individual homes to develop their own particular ethos and approach to care' (Department of Health 2002b: 3), in practice, the framework offers little opportunity for staff initiative, intellect or creativity. At the same time, it places an emphasis on inspection and a demand for documented evidence of adherence to procedure that was criticised by many English respondents as adding to their workload, at the expense of time spent 'being together' with young people. In this strongly procedural approach, the worker's role is focused on child protection, not child development. Her (his) function is constrained by an emphasis on ensuring security and safety, rather like the role of a warden or a minder, a maintaining rather than a developmental role, less concerned with the 'upbringing' of the child in a pedagogic sense.

This characterisation precludes a fully professional role for the English care worker: (s)he does not have the education, the autonomy, or the status in relation to other professionals. In contrast, the social pedagogue can be seen as an 'active agent of care', in residential settings where the work is conceptualised in terms of supporting holistic development[6], rather than in terms of 'holding' or behaviour management. The social pedagogue works alongside and with the whole young person and their networks on all dimensions of their lives, working with heart, hands, and head – with emotions, practical projects and theories – in a multi-dimensional way (see Figure 6.1). A Danish student who took part in the first phase of our research spoke of having a 'professional heart'. By this, she meant that while one did not have to like all the young people, one had to be prepared to use the self to 'gain access to their way of thinking and feeling.' This approach was most evident in Danish workers' accounts of their practice; for German

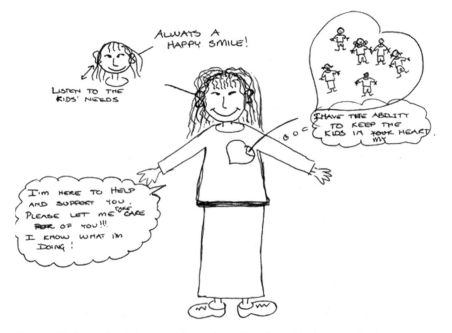

Figure 6.1 A 'good pedagogue' (drawn by a Danish student).

social pedagogues the discourse around social pedagogy seemed rather less extensive, and practice perhaps more uneven, possibly reflecting the higher level of qualification among Danish residential care workers.

A considerable number of professionals are involved with young people looked after in residential care. In England, for example, this may include the child's social worker (or, out of office hours, the emergency duty social worker); officers of the Children and Family Court Advisory and Support Service (CAFCASS) and of the Care Standards Commission; a solicitor or advocate; and for older young people, a personal advisor appointed under the Children (Leaving Care) Act (2002). Many English interviewees expressed frustration about the division of responsibility between the variety of individuals involved in decisions about young people and their care. In part this related to the perceived low status of residential care work in England, such that workers and managers felt they had a diminished voice in decision making.[7] Such difficulties were rarely mentioned by Danish respondents, and only slightly more often by German care workers. Division of responsibility for different areas of the child's life was also reflected in the lower proportion of English workers involved in liaison with other professionals (52 per cent in England; 67 per cent in Germany; and 66 per cent in Denmark). Teamwork and multidisciplinary working are key elements of the social pedagogic approach, and form part of the professional education; at the same time, the professional status of social pedagogues may give them a stronger 'voice' than their English care workers in discussions with colleagues from other professional disciplines such as field social work.

English workers were also less likely to be involved in liaison with children's families (33 per cent) than those in Germany (48 per cent) or Denmark (71 per cent). This may partly reflect role divisions such as those indicated above, if family liaison in England is primarily the responsibility of the child's social worker, but it also reflects a differing approach to care between the countries. Social pedagogy's holistic principles dictate that close collaborative links should be maintained with parents and other family members throughout a young person's placement, and social pedagogues learn ways of working with families during their professional education.

Future directions

So, what does professionalisation bring to residential care work? Our research suggests there are benefits for employers in Denmark and Germany, where residential home managers reported lower levels of staff turnover, with few recruitment or retention difficulties. At the same time, Danish and, to a slightly lesser extent, German workers appeared to feel more satisfied and valued in the work they do, and better able to withstand 'the rigours of the job' than their English colleagues. The social pedagogic approach also appears to make a difference to the practice of care work: this was evident in the workers' accounts of their practice and of the young people in their care. Undoubtedly, social pedagogues benefit in many ways from their professional status, and the resources offered by their professional education. It must be recognised, however, that the differences we have described in workforce and practice issues are not simply about professionality, or social pedagogic education, but are rooted in the policy and wider cultural context of the countries studied.

Pedagogy, as it is understood in continental Europe, provides a coherent and well-established discourse underpinning policy and practice for all children, including those looked after, within the countries in which we conducted our research. In relation to residential care, social pedagogic policies are often based on what is seen as the 'emancipation' of young people, through the broad objectives of 'promoting individuals' and developing their independence. These principles are reflected in policy requirements for young people's participation in decisions and plans for their care. In Denmark, for example, children aged 15 years and over should agree to and jointly develop plans for their care. In Germany, policy based on the need for individual care plans and for a *Lebensweltorientierung* (literally, a 'living world orientation') has led to a diversification of placement possibilities, with policy support for the establishment of small local facilities, and of different forms of residential institution, such as 'five day settings'. Importantly, in these countries, these policies have led to the conceptualisation of residential care as a positive placement choice for young people, an opportunity for therapeutic and developmental intervention, rather than as a final option when other possibilities are exhausted. It is instructive that, unlike respondents in England, staff and managers in Germany and Denmark did not mention adverse comment in the mass media about the status of their work or the performance of residential care, in a way that might question the role of the sector in caring for looked-after children.

The contrasting construction of residential care provision as a place of protection and containment for young people, with corresponding implications for the workers' role, is not unique to England. Indeed, it has much in common with historical accounts of the development of residential care in the countries studied, as they have moved from ideas of custody, reform and supervision towards pedagogic models, with an emphasis on therapeutic work geared towards upbringing (education-in-its-broadest-sense) of young people, with a positive value given to supporting their holistic development. Perhaps in England, residential care work simply is at an earlier stage in this developmental process.

Although the professionalisation of the workforce and the development of education is less advanced in England than in the other countries studied, education of the English care workforce and the creation of a more coherent framework of qualifications are government priorities for social care. This is evident in the work of the national Training Organisation for the Personal Social Services (TOPSS), and within key policy documents concerned with children and young people, such as *Every Child Matters* (Department for

Education and Skills 2003) and the Children Act (2004). These contain ideas and recommendations that accord with social pedagogic principles, such as 'educating through and for society and communities' (Hämäläinen 2003: 73).

Our research suggests that residential care work in England would benefit from the professionalisation of the workforce through a social pedagogic education. In the words of Moyles (2001), 'for practice to meet professional status, both head and heart need to meet at the interface of reflection' (90). Undoubtedly, it would prove challenging to introduce the social pedagogic model of training and education to England, so as to create a professional care worker within the current policy and practice context. Social pedagogues would have little opportunity to apply their reflexive professional skills and judgement, given the present procedure-bound regulatory framework in English residential care. At the same time, the present workforce, with its varied, low-level and technically based qualifications, probably needs the strictures of current legislation to achieve accountability and consistency of practice across the sector, qualities that, we would argue, are enabled by the generalist professional education that is social pedagogy, with its emphasis on reflection, respect for the child, and discussion of practice.

Ultimately, social pedagogy is more than a profession or a model for training. It is a whole way of conceptualising work that encompasses care but much else besides: pedagogical work takes us beyond care work. Hämäläinen (2003: 72) described the nature, range and scope of social pedagogy as 'both problematic and inspiring', and this is certainly true of its potential application to policy and practice for children and young people in England. The benefits indicated by our research lead us to conclude that the value of a professional educated workforce warrants the challenge of establishing a social pedagogic approach to care work for the future.

Notes

1 This is a composite portrait, based on a number of interviews. Mette is a pseudonym.
2 For the purposes of this chapter, we will use the terms 'social pedagogy' and 'social pedagogues' to refer to this continental European model of training and practice, and to make clear its distinction from the English language conceptualisation of pedagogy as formal education.
3 As discussed in chapter 4, UK policy has also prioritised the creation of a coherent framework for training the care workforce, but the current approach to training remains fragmentary, based on a variety of vocational qualifications. This training is predominantly task and workplace based, focused on occupation-specific competencies, and as such is quite different in nature from the continental European discipline of social pedagogy, with its origins in critical educational theory (Hämäläinen 2003).
4 In England, the term 'looked after' was introduced by the Children Act (1989) to refer to children and young people who are 'accommodated by the local authority'

for more than 24 hours, either with parental agreement, or subject to a Care Order passed by a court, or at the request of the young person (over the age of 16). For simplicity, this term will be used in reference to children 'in care' in all the countries that were part of our research.

5   Source of Looked After Children statistics. England: Department for Education and Skills, figures for year ending 31 March 2003. Denmark: Statbank Denmark, figures for year ending 31 December 2003. Germany: Federal Statistical Office: Fachserie 13, Reihe 6.1.2, Reihe, 6.1.4: Jugendhilfe – Erzieherische Hilfen außerhalb des Elternhauses, 1998.

6   For example, Nohl (1935, cited in Hämäläinen, 2003), who developed the first professional education for social pedagogues in Germany, envisaged social pedagogy as an holistic approach to understanding clients and their situations as a whole, in terms of human action in historical, psychological, cultural and social spheres.

7   English residential care workers' perception that they lack a voice in decision making is borne out by documentation such as the Pathway Plans (Department of Health 2003) required for young people leaving care, under the Children (Leaving Care) Act. The related paperwork requires signatures from those who have agreed the Pathway Plan, including the young person, parents, personal advisor and social worker, but not the residential care worker.

7 Mentors for children and young people who offend, or are at risk of offending

An emerging profession?

Ginny Greenlaw and Ian St James Roberts

Margaret is 31 years old, employed as a full-time care worker, and became a mentor after seeing an advertisement in a local newspaper. The mentor project on which she worked offered training and a National Vocational Qualification, and Margaret was attracted to the idea of adding to her professional credentials. At her interview, Margaret said that she also liked the idea of helping young people who were getting into trouble, partly because her own adolescence had been difficult, and she had been helped greatly by a teacher who had gone out of her way to provide guidance and support. By becoming a mentor, Margaret hoped to give something back to the community.

After training with the mentor project over two Saturdays, Margaret was matched with Peter, a 16-year-old whose father is in prison, and who has a poor relationship with his mother. He has not attended school since he was excluded a year ago for persistent truanting and behaviour problems. He had gained no qualifications at school and was told he had learning difficulties. He had been arrested for car theft and joy riding on several occasions. The local Youth Offending Team had referred Peter to the mentor project.

Margaret was told by the mentor project that her first goal was to establish trust and rapport between Peter and herself. They had met for two hours on Saturdays, first at a local café and then to share activities such as bowling. Margaret's first challenge, she quickly discovered, was to get Peter to turn up: he had repeatedly failed to do so. He also lacked any social graces, was often surly, and seemed to have difficulty in concentrating and communicating his thoughts. Peter did eventually tell her that, following a row with his mother, he had moved out of her flat. By contacting housing agencies and social services, Margaret was able to find him some accommodation. This gained her some credit with Peter and he had begun to open up to her. After discussion with the mentor project, Margaret had begun helping Peter to put together a written CV and to complete the application forms for a local college. She hoped to persuade him to take a training course in car mechanics, which would match his interest in cars.

The word 'mentor' comes originally from the Greek poet Homer's tale *The Odyssey* (Homer 800 BC). While he was fighting the Trojan War, Ulysses appointed a family friend, called Mentor, to be tutor-advisor to his son and guardian of his estates. In more current usage, the on-line *Oxford English Dictionary* defines a 'mentor' as 'a person who acts as guide and adviser to another person, especially one who is younger and less experienced'. 'Mentoring' is 'the activity of a mentor' and 'the action of advising or training another person, especially a less experienced colleague'. Mentoring of this sort has become popular over the last decade in many regions of the world, including Europe (ENYMO 2004) North America (Grossman and Tierney 1998) and Australia (ARTD 2002).

Mentoring relationships can exist informally, as in the case of Margaret's relationship with a teacher, described above. However, the interest here is in formal mentor programmes, which have been set up deliberately with a purpose in mind. In these instances, a mentor is supervised by a mentor project, which has responsibility for mentor training and for supporting and managing the mentor programme, which the mentor delivers to the young person or 'mentee'. In particular, the focus here is on mentor programmes that have been set up to help children and young people who are getting into trouble with the law. Mentoring for this purpose is now being widely adopted both as a component of professional development and as an important part of efforts to address the problems of social exclusion and vulnerable youth (Rhodes et al. 2002).

The use of mentor programmes to support and redirect the development of young people who have committed criminal offences, or are likely to do so, raises special, and substantial, challenges. This chapter is based on our experience in evaluating mentor projects for the UK Home Office and Youth Justice Board for England and Wales (YJB)[1], which will be referred to as the 'Mentoring' study (St James-Roberts et al. 2004a). The chapter will first review the emerging evidence about the effectiveness of mentoring in helping such young people. We will draw a distinction between 'non-directive' mentor programmes and those that seek to impart competencies to the young people involved. In the second part of the chapter, we will propose the need to develop a more formalised, competency-focused, form of mentoring as a new type of profession. The guiding or broadly educational orientation of mentoring may have parallels with forms of care work discussed elsewhere in this volume, particularly the work of pedagogues in residential care (chapter 6).

Emerging knowledge about the effectiveness of mentor programmes

Reasons for the appeal of mentoring

Youth mentoring emerged in North America in 1904, with the Big Brothers Big Sisters scheme (http://www.bbbsa.org) which aimed to provide supportive adult friends to young people. However, a widespread increase in the use of mentoring to address social exclusion and disaffected youth has been a feature of the last 10–15 years. In England, several mentor projects emerged in the 1990s including the Dalston Youth Project and Project CHANCE (St James-Roberts and Singh 2001; Tarling et al. 2001). Between 1999 and 2002, the YJB funded 43 mentoring projects (Tarling et al. 2004) and the government in England introduced several intervention schemes that included mentoring as a component part. For instance, Connexions schemes, which support people aged 13 to 19 in making a smooth transition to adulthood and working life, provide community mentors and personal advisers as an integral part of their service (Connexions Service National Unit and the Youth Justice Board 2001). More recently, the YJB has committed just under 12 million pounds over three years to fund 84 new projects to provide mentors to young people who offend, or are at risk of offending.

The increasing popularity of youth mentoring probably reflects social and political pressures that are common to many modern societies. First, the widely publicised perception that crime is rife, together with evidence that offending patterns of behaviour are often established at an early age (Farrington 1996; Loeber 1990), has focused attention on the underlying reasons and need for remedies. Second, the belief that the breakdown of family and community values is responsible has led governments to invest in initiatives designed to increase social cohesion and 'social capital', that is, the relationships between people and organisations within a community which theorists view as its social 'glue' (Halpern 2003). To some extent, the popularity of mentoring reflects an attempt to compensate for deficiencies within society that are thought to put children and young people at risk (Rhodes et al. 2002).

Against this background, mentor projects are only one type of initiative, schemes designed to improve parenting skills being another example (Ghate and Ramella 2002). The appeal of mentor projects, in particular, lies in their community basis and potential cost-effectiveness. An almost universal feature of mentor projects that target disaffected youth is that the mentors are community volunteers. As a result, YJB mentor projects, for example, help to meet government targets for community enhancement by increasing the number of community volunteers. Although mentor projects usually employ salaried staff to manage mentors, the volunteer status of most mentors makes this approach to crime reduction potentially cheap. Indeed, the metric by which success is judged is often not effectiveness, but cost-effectiveness, since a less effective, but cheaper, method can be more cost-effective. It follows that mentor programmes need not work on every occasion; the acid test is whether they are more cost effective than other options.

The features of successful mentor programmes

In spite of the rapid expansion of mentor projects for young people at risk, there are still remarkably few systematic evaluations of their results. One reason for this is that the outcome of such projects, reduction in rates of offending, requires evidence to be accumulated across large numbers and over the long term, while mentor projects, and studies of them, are conducted over the short term with relatively small numbers. A related complication is how to measure offending and its reduction, since the existing methods all have weaknesses. These issues are examined in more detail elsewhere (Farrington 1989; Graham and Bowling 1995).

The upshot of these provisos is that it is not yet possible to provide an evidence-based answer to the question 'what works?' Instead, what has emerged from the recent literature are distinctions that point to the sorts of features which are necessary for successful delivery of mentor programmes, together with some indications as to what works at least some of the time. Below, we will try to summarise the main themes and findings, and indicate the main areas of controversy emerging from recent research. As well as drawing on our own and others' experience in evaluating mentor projects, we will take account of lessons learned from broader evaluations of what works in preventing offending, such as Lipsey's (1995) meta-analysis of 400 intervention studies.

Successfully involving the targeted young people

Both our own and others' studies of mentor projects provide evidence that young offenders, children and adolescents with behaviour problems, school truanting and exclusion, and other factors that increase the probability of offending, can be recruited successfully by mentor projects (Shiner et al. 2004). Taking our evaluation of 84 mentor projects spread across England and Wales as an example (St James-Roberts et al. 2004b), the projects enrolled 2,843 mentees between the age of 10 and 17 during the first two years of their three-year funding. Over half of the young people were referred to the mentor projects by Youth Offending Teams (YOTs)[2], and others by statutory or voluntary organisations for at-risk young people and by schools. Three-quarters had a known history of offending and many were on a referral order, supervision order, final warning, or detention and training order. The young people had high rates of truanting and exclusion from school and 51 per cent had literacy needs, 48 per cent numeracy needs, 28 per cent special educational needs, and 16 per cent had statements for special educational needs. Similarly, the recent evaluation of ten 'Mentoring Plus' projects carried out for the Joseph Rowntree Foundation (Shiner et al. 2004), found that 400 young people had been recruited and assigned mentors. Here, too, many had been referred by Youth Offending Teams, offending levels were high, truancy and exclusion rates were greatly above community norms, and many had a history of severely disrupted school and family lives.

As well as recruiting the targeted young people, mentor projects have to engage and maintain them in their mentor programmes. Here, the findings are more mixed, with substantial variations between projects, indicating that some have more successful strategies for delivering their mentor programmes than others. Shiner et al. (2004) found that 57 per cent of the young people recruited by Mentoring Plus actually took part in mentoring on a monthly basis or more often, while our interim figures from the YJB projects are of a similar order (St James-Roberts et al. 2004b). Whether these figures are considered promising or disappointing depends very much on how they are viewed. First, they are not poor compared to those from other types of community intervention projects targeting similar young people (Ghate and Ramella 2002). Second, bearing in mind the multiply disadvantaged backgrounds of these socially disaffected young people, it could well be argued that delivering a mentor programme to half of them is a major achievement. Third, their immediate implication is that variations between projects are probably more important than average figures. Realistically, it is unlikely that all mentor programmes will succeed with all young people – it is more likely that some programmes will be effective in some cases. It follows that the immediate goal is to identify the features of those mentor projects and programmes that work effectively, and to understand why. For this purpose, the findings so far look promising.

As well as suiting programmes to the needs of young people, a second issue is whether particular sub-groups of young people benefit especially from mentor programmes. Recent Youth Justice Board mentor projects, for instance, have targeted groups with literacy and numeracy difficulties, as well as groups from minority ethnic backgrounds. Other variables of this sort include age – in the belief that children will respond better to mentors than adolescents – and whether young people who take part voluntarily fare better than those who are coerced to do so. Evidence about these issues is currently lacking.

The characteristics of mentors

Since the young people recruited by mentor projects in this area have multiple disadvantages and are socially alienated, they present obvious challenges for community volunteers seeking to gain their trust and help them to change their lives. The debate about what makes a mentor successful has revolved around three main mentor characteristics: demographic background, personal characteristics, and training.

There is evidence that mentors' demographic features, including gender, ethnicity, cultural background, and religious persuasion, influence mentees and their families at the outset, so that some families refuse to accept possible mentors who do not match the mentee in these respects (St James-Roberts and Singh 2001). To some extent, this is consistent with the widespread view of mentors as role models, that is, as someone like the mentee who can provide a mature example of success. In practice, this does create some problems, since virtually all mentor projects receive far more applications from women than men to be mentors, while the vast majority of mentees are male. In recent YJB mentor projects, for example, 66 per cent of trained mentors were women, while 76 per cent of mentees were young men. Some projects have had similar difficulty in recruiting mentors with minority ethnic, cultural and religious backgrounds.

Although this problem needs to be recognised, its importance should not be exaggerated. Examples exist of mentor projects which have succeeded in matching ethnicity (Tarling et al. 2001), so that here, too, successful strategies need to be understood and built upon. Indeed, the question of how to recruit and match mentors with mentees is a broader one, with a range of practices apparent among mentor projects. In most cases, the projects carry out the matching, but some allow the mentor (or mentee) to choose who they are matched with, sometimes following a 'residential', where mentees and their potential mentors have got to know each other (Shiner et al. 2004; Tarling et al. 2001). At the moment, we do not know whether any of these variations has a substantial effect on the outcomes of mentor programmes, while the evidence to date is that most mentees and their families value the personal characteristics of mentors more than their broad, social-demographic features (St James-Roberts and Singh 2001). Clearly, some families' requirement for demographic matching needs to be recognised and accommodated by mentor projects, since otherwise they will not be able to deliver some mentor programmes. However, there is a need, too, for evidence that matched mentor programmes produce more successful outcomes than programmes set up in other ways, and which identifies the most effective methods of matching. Evidence on these issues is sparse.

When asked about their expectations of mentors, most mentees and parents who participated in the evaluation of project CHANCE stated that they had few preconceptions, except that the mentor would provide support (St James-Roberts and Singh 2001). The mentor's commitment to helping the mentee, and ability to do so, were more important in most cases than her, or his, ethnicity, gender, or religion. This finding emphasises the need to look beyond broad descriptors, to identify the personal features that make some mentors particularly successful. It may be that this kind of commitment is similar to the ethic of care or habit of mind discussed in chapter 1.

Since trust is a defining feature of mentor–mentee relationships, a mentor's ability to establish this is a key requirement, which most mentors have been found to possess. All the studies that have examined this have found that the vast majority of mentors are trusted and valued by their mentees (Shiner et al. 2004; St James-Roberts and Singh 2001; VTO 2000). A second key variable is motivational commitment, since many mentors report that mentoring is an uphill struggle, particularly in the early stages of the relationship, when ground rules are being established (Colley 2003). The chief reasons given by mentors for wanting to make this commitment are the need to 'give something back' to society, often because they have received such help themselves in the past, and the need to accumulate experience and qualifications towards their own careers (St James-Roberts and Singh 2001). These motivations are similar to the reasons given by other groups of care workers for taking up their work (Cameron et al. 2001; Petrie et al. forthcoming). It is not clear whether one or other of these reasons is more important in maintaining motivation and both may well have a part to play.

It is sometimes said that mentors need to have a particular type of personality and that good mentors are born, not bred, much as good teachers are believed to be. This idea has commonalities with the notion of an ethic of care; an emphasis on personal qualities as a basis for care work can also be seen in the descriptions of English workers in children's residential care in chapter 6. If true, this proposal could be helpful, so far as it leads to methods of screening and identification, which would allow good mentors to be recruited. To the best of our knowledge, this has not been achieved, so that the reasons for screening out would-be mentors revolve around unsuitability, for instance because of a police record, and applicants' commitment throughout the selection and training process. One controversial issue is whether reformed criminals make the best mentors, because of their insight and mentees' identification with them. This is an intriguing question, but it does not seem to have been put to the test. Clearly, more studies of personal attributes that suit individuals to being mentors are needed but, in our view, are unlikely to be productive in the short term, since few mentor projects are currently so overwhelmed with applicant mentors that they can afford to turn many away. For both practical and ideological reasons, the need for better mentor training and management is the immediate priority. Because these aspects of mentor effectiveness are primarily the responsibility of mentor projects, we will discuss them below. A recommended source for mentors who wish to avoid many of the pitfalls involved in programme delivery is 'Twelve Habits of the Toxic Mentor' (Clutterbuck 2001).

The integrity of mentor projects

Projects select mentors and mentees, then train, support and monitor mentors while they deliver mentor programmes, and are responsible for the policies, infrastructure and networks with other organisations that underpin mentoring. Because mentoring as a formal intervention is still finding its feet, it is not surprising that evaluations so far have found that some projects fail to become established, or to deliver viable numbers of mentor programmes (ARTD 2002). It is important to recognise that these pitfalls are not specific to mentor projects, but rather are shared by community intervention projects in general (Hine and Harrington 2004). Fortunately, the features of project integrity associated with effective delivery have begun to emerge. Below, we will summarise these features and indicate some of the associated issues and controversies.

Effective networking, administration and record-keeping

Although some projects fail to become established because they cannot recruit enough mentors or mentees, the main reason for their failure, in our experience, is weakness in project administration and networking with other organisations. It is difficult to establish effective liaison with other agencies, particularly where these are statutory services such as Youth Offending Teams and schools. Professional barriers, confidentiality issues, and the pressures under which modern statutory services operate, all conspire to make things difficult for voluntary community projects. These challenges are greater where projects are managed by community volunteers, who may not be trained or experienced in the necessary skills, and where projects have a limited time to become established, because of the short-term funding that characterises many mentor projects to date. In turn, this leads to rapid staff turnover, and associated loss of network contacts. As a result, mentor projects are seldom operating under optimum conditions, as they would be if properly integrated within statutory community services. It follows that evaluations probably underestimate their potential.

Mentor projects' first goal is to help the young people they are responsible for, so that the added burdens of administration and record-keeping are seldom priorities, particularly when staffing and funding are limited, as is the case with most mentor projects evaluated to date. Fortunately, many projects provide an indication of the sorts of administrative structures needed in order to deliver mentor programmes successfully. The following are the key features emerging in recent research:

- Effective collection of background information about the mentee, so that a mentor programme can be tailored to his individual need.
- Mentor training that is perceived to be effective by mentors and others involved.
- Regular monitoring and supervision of mentors, together with target-setting and record-keeping that is administered by the project. A common problem is that mentors are left to their own devices. Projects need to monitor that the programme delivered reflects their policies, that changes are occurring and recorded by mentors, and that targets are reviewed and updated by the project.

- Preparation for the end of mentoring. Unless the goal of a mentor programme is clearly defined and recognised, there is a danger that mentees will feel abandoned and let down when the programme ends. In contrast, mentor programmes which end when their goals are achieved, are clearly marked by a 'graduation' or other celebratory occasion, and this leads to a planned next stage, allow mentees to feel a sense of achievement and to move on in their lives.
- The need for a plausible, clearly articulated theory of change. The lack of a clearly worked out rationale for why an intervention programme should work is a common weakness among community-based projects (Connell et al. 1995), and a stumbling block for some mentor projects. The central question is how a mentor relationship can change an at-risk young person in a way that leads him away from offending. More precisely, does the relationship change the mentee, and in what way should this reduce risk? Having a plausible, fully articulated theory of this kind does not guarantee success, but the lack of a theory makes the intervention unfocused.

The scope and goals of mentor programmes

The most common form of mentor programme is a one-to-one relationship, such that a mentor and mentee meet for a few hours about once per week, to share activities designed to cement their relationship and establish compatibility and trust. Often, this involves walking and talking together, and sports and other recreational activities, including visits to cinemas and cafes (VTO 2000). In effect, these are the sorts of activities young people do with friends and with their families.

Although this remains the dominant model of mentoring, the recent YJB mentor initiative has deliberately sought to enhance mentees' literacy and numeracy abilities as a major goal. Of 84 projects funded, 53 set out to recruit young people whose histories both put them at risk of future offending and who had literacy or numeracy difficulties. Other projects have targeted competencies that involve basic literacy skills, such as the ability to read and fill in forms, work out timetables, and to put together a CV. Others again have focused on the use of computers and acquisition of computer skills, or participation in health education or anger management programmes. The common denominator is to increase competencies that enable the young person to engage with social, educational and employment environments, which in turn will foster their development.

As well as varying in the targets of mentor programmes, the 84 projects vary greatly in how the programmes are delivered. In some of them, mentors themselves deliver sessions designed to enhance mentees' literacy, numeracy or other skills, while other projects employ separate business and student mentors, or other multiple mentor arrangements. Some, like the original Dalston Youth Project discussed earlier in this chapter (Tarling et al. 2001), have separate mentors and tutors who work together. Most mentoring is carried out on a one-to-one basis in the community, but a few projects deliver mentoring on the project premises, some deliver mentoring in a group setting, and one combines these procedures, with each mentee allocated to one mentor and all of them sitting together around one large table. In a few cases, members of the project team have delivered mentoring so that they are, in effect, employed as paid mentors. The following thumbnail sketches for three of the mentor projects included in the current YJB mentor scheme provide some idea of the diversity that exists among contemporary mentor programmes.

Three different mentor projects within the current Youth Justice Board scheme: accounts extracted from project records.

Project 1 is based in the North West of England. It targets young people from Black and minority ethnic or hard-to-reach communities, most of whom are over the age of 15. It is an independent organisation with formal links with the local Youth Offending Team, as well strong links with the local Volunteer Bureau, schools and social services departments. Mentors are given one full day of mentoring awareness training, together with the opportunity to do an Open College Network qualification in mentoring. Some mentors take a basic skills awareness training course, which explores how to deliver basic literacy and numeracy skills, while some complete City and Guilds Initial Certificate in Teaching Basic Skills (Literacy) 9282. Mentor training is provided both in-house, by the project and through links with local colleges and community agencies. The generic mentoring training is run in partnership with the local probation service.

Mentoring programmes: Each young person has one mentor with whom they meet weekly for a 6–12 month period in a community setting. Mentoring also prioritises social skills, life skills and 'advocacy', which aims to put the young person in touch with community services. Programmes designed to improve mentees' literacy and numeracy skills are delivered by a tutor and by some mentors who have completed the 9282 qualification. Young people can spend up to two half-days per week on literacy and numeracy programmes, according to need. The majority of young people attend mentoring on a voluntary basis but, in about 10 per cent of cases, YOT case managers have made mentoring part of a Court Order.

Project's account of difficulties and successes: 'Problems have arisen due to the diversity of the young people – some had no interest in education and it was hard work to engage them and their parents. However, on the positive side, some young people have re-engaged into school, and some have completed work experience, college courses and gone into employment. The project has been bombarded with referrals and could never offer enough spaces to keep up with demand.'

Project 2 is a numeracy and literacy-focused project based in the South East of England. It is part of a larger charity and has formal links with the local Youth Offending Team and strong working links with the County Council, Under 19 Substance Misuse Team, the Youth Development Service and the police. The project provides its mentors with two weeks of training in-house. It targets people between the ages of 14 and 17.

Mentoring programmes: Mentoring is carried out on a one-to-one basis, but in a group setting, such that the young people sit round one large table with individual mentors. The mentee attends the project four afternoons a week for the duration of the programme, which varies in length according to the needs and preferences of the young person. Most mentoring activities are held on the project premises, but there are also external activities, such as working on a farm for a day. Numeracy and literacy programmes are delivered by the mentor for at least 10 hours per week. Mentoring also aims to promote life and social skills, and includes advocacy work. Originally, all the young people took part in mentoring as part of their Court Order, but now mentoring occurs more often without an order.

Project's account of difficulties and successes: 'An initial difficulty was getting people to acknowledge that the mentees were out of education. However, there have some real successes. One is a young man for whom an award ceremony was organised because, having experienced quite an ordeal, he sat a Higher Diploma in Music Technology and Sound Engineering. Various young people have returned to college or school – even though they were complete non-attendees beforehand. Many young people have passed City and Guilds exams, and there have been successes in reducing re-offending. This is a well-known project in the community, and the project provides feedback to a steering group representing lots of agencies.'

Project 3 is a numeracy and literacy-focused mentor project based in Wales. It is part of a safer city charity. Mentors are given a two-day training course run in-house by the mentor project. The project works

closely with a local school in a deprived area of the city, so that 11- to-
13-year-olds who are at risk of offending are referred to the project by
their Head of Year.

Mentoring programmes: Each young person has one mentor with
whom they meet for 12 weeks in a community setting. Mentoring is
issue-based, including social and life skills, as well as literacy and
numeracy abilities. The project always sends mentees on external
courses, which typically involve three full days of outdoor activities
designed to enhance team building. A specialist tutor delivers the
numeracy/literacy support, so that once a week, the young people
spend two hours in tutoring and then two hours with their mentor. The
young people attend mentoring on a voluntary basis but encouraged
by their school.

Project's account of difficulties and successes: 'The main difficulty
has been with funding. The project has been very successful and the
school is very supportive. The project has definitely led to a reduction
in non-attendance and to improvements in behaviour.'

Purists might dispute whether some of the interventions described above
really count as mentoring, but this would be to miss the point. Mentor
programmes have already evolved and are likely to continue to do so, as the
most effective strategies emerge. Moreover, many ordinary friendships
involve sharing knowledge and skills, whether this involves learning the
rules of card games or sports, or sharing of the more formal skills needed to
read a map or use the Internet. The boundaries between friendships and
learning relationships are inherently fuzzy and permeable, just as former
distinctions between education and care have begun to be bridged in New
Zealand and some European countries, leading to the hybrid sometimes
called 'educare' (DfES 2004). Indeed, even the original Mentor was tutor, as
well as advisor, to Ulysses' son. Instead of debating the true nature of mentoring, it is more important to establish what works, under what circumstances, and why. An important emerging distinction is between mentor
programmes which are 'non-directive' and seek only to befriend a young
person and those that we will call 'competency-focused'; that is, they set out
to improve the mentee's psychological, social or other skills, in order to
change his interactions with other people and the physical world. This
distinction echoes questions raised in chapter 1 about the aims and
value-base of care work, for example in relation to Roche and Rankin's
(2004) definition of care work achieving 'social inclusion and better life
opportunities for vulnerable people'.

For instance, in her review of the Big Brothers Big Sisters (BBBS) project,
McGill (1999) emphasised that the BBBS aim was simply to provide mentees

with a supportive adult friend, rather than to provide a directive influence. At least on the face of it, however, it is hard to understand why a friendship with an older person, in and of itself, would have a positive influence on a young person, since there is evidence that friendships with other at-risk people can increase the risk of offending (Graham and Bowling 1995), while at least one evaluation has found some mentoring friendships to be harmful (O'Donnell et al. 1979). It is possible to articulate how an adult friend might induce change, for instance by making a young person change his attitudes and behaviours to match those of a valued model, but so far no theory of this kind has been put forward or tested, so far as we know.

Rather than mentoring that is based solely on befriending, the alternative – a competency-focused form of mentor programme – has its origins in projects such as the Dalston Youth Project and Project CHANCE (St James-Roberts and Singh 2001; Tarling et al. 2001). Both of these approaches sought to enhance child or youth competencies, in the case of the Dalston 'Mentoring Plus' project by supplementing the mentor programme with direct educational instruction from teachers. This particular approach is interesting, in that it aims to reduce some risk factors known to predict offending, but an obvious objection is that it only adds insult to injury. That is, given that the young people participating have already truanted or been excluded from school, why should they respond positively to 'more of the same'? A different, but equally telling objection is that mentors are not teachers, while it is difficult to see how community volunteers could acquire the sorts of skills needed via the limited training that most mentor projects can provide.

These criticisms imply the need for some substantial re-thinking about the development of mentoring programmes. On one hand, there is a need to develop strategies that can bridge care and education, so that disaffected young people elect to take part in activities which are educational in a broad, rather than narrow, sense. On the other hand, there is a need for clarity about the scope and role of mentors, relative to other professional and voluntary agencies who provide disaffected young people with support. If mentors are to do more than befriend, what sorts of competencies should they focus on and what form should the resulting mentor programme take? For instance, should mentors be facilitators, who put mentees in touch with separate educational, health and other community services, or should they aim to help young people develop some basic competencies themselves? Between them, the 84 YJB projects in the Mentoring Study under evaluation include both these and other alternatives.

In concluding this part of the chapter, it is clear that mentoring as a form of provision for young people who offend or are at risk of offending is still finding its feet. Some central principles for successful projects and programme delivery have begun to emerge, and it is striking that the lessons learned bear a close resemblance to the findings from evaluations of crime-reduction interventions more generally. Lipsey's (1995) meta-analysis, for example, concluded that project integrity and a clear focus on the development of participants' skills and competencies, were key features of successful crime reduction programmes.

A danger for a fledgling provision like mentoring is that it might be dismissed prematurely, before its promise has been properly examined. For example, a recent review both pointed to the dearth of evidence that non-directive mentoring is effective and recommended that other forms of intervention, such as cognitive-behaviour therapy, should be adopted instead (Roberts et al. 2004). Although this conclusion was confined to non-directive mentor programmes, this distinction may be overlooked, while the urgent wish for solutions may drive policy in other directions without due reason. The evidence available about alternatives to mentoring, such as cognitive-behaviour therapy and parenting programmes, is also very limited and it is becoming clear that each of these approaches has important limitations (Spencer 2003). Rather than rolling out any one approach for routine adoption, it may be more fruitful to develop and build on the promising features of each approach. In the rest of this chapter, we will argue that a more professionalised version of mentoring that achieves this can provide a blueprint for the future.

Mentoring: a blueprint for an emerging profession?

As well as the changes that are taking place in the form and contents of mentoring, a striking feature of its recent history is its increasing professionalisation. Mentors can study for and gain National Vocational Qualifications (NVQs) Open College Network (OCN), or other college or even university qualifications. Based on government-sponsored Education Business Partnerships, the Department for Education and Skills' Excellence in Mentoring Award provides schools with a framework for accreditation of effective mentor schemes. Together, these and other developments are likely to attract more participants and sustain their involvement whilst increasing public confidence and raising the professional profile of mentor programmes. If the qualifications lead to professional status and salaries, some of the difficulties which currently face mentor projects, including the shortage of male mentors, may also be resolved.

Mentoring is not the only emerging blueprint for future forms of social care for young people who offend or are at risk of offending. In 2003, the Institute for Public Policy Research concluded

> that new types of professionals are needed who can apply a range of skills and knowledge when working with young people. These will be people who can gain the trust and confidence of a young person and have a range of options available to support them. If the focus of youth work is primarily on increasing educational achievement or on providing diversionary activities to keep young people out of trouble there is a

danger that the underlying causes of low expectations and problem behaviour are not tackled head on. A new profession might combine youth and community work, social work, adolescent mental health services and careers services to provide more holistic services for young people. This is a role that is filled to an extent by social educators on the continent.

(Edwards and Hatch 2003)

The term 'social educators' here shares much of its meaning with the word 'pedagogue', as it is used elsewhere in this book (see, for example, chapter 6). Another, similar, professional category beginning to emerge is that of 'advocates' (YJB 2004), while English government schemes such as the Connexions service include a variety of professionals who help 13–19-year-olds to make the transition to adulthood. Since there is clearly a degree of overlap between these different role categories, it may be helpful to clarify the key features that distinguish mentoring programmes.

From the Mentoring study, four important characteristics of mentors have been identified. First, mentors represent the young person they are supporting and have no direct statutory authority, responsibilities, or powers. They are 'on the young person's side' and represent his or her interests. To paraphrase one mother of a Project CHANCE mentee, the mentor 'had not come to take her son away' (St James-Roberts and Singh 2001). At a time when social workers, probation officers, and others involved with young offenders are increasingly taken up with 'administrative surveillance and control' (Barry 2000), mentors focus on the needs and wishes of young people.

The second defining feature of mentoring, which arguably follows from the first, is the mentee's trust in the mentor. Some mentor projects deliberately set out to build a trusting relationship as the first step in the mentor programme, only introducing other targets once this has been achieved.

A third feature is the unequal nature of the relationship, such that a more knowledgeable, usually more mature, mentor befriends and helps a young person.

A fourth characteristic, following the arguments put forward here, is that the mentor seeks to impart competencies that help the young person to engage more effectively with his or her environment. As noted above, these may be basic social and life skills, as well as more complex abilities.

The challenge for the future is how to maintain these four attributes and to combine them with emerging knowledge about other features of intervention programmes that produce positive results. One way to do so might be to provide mentoring with a professional status, together with the training, accreditation and formal links with other statutory and community agencies which that involves. The price of developing mentoring in this way could be to lose the community volunteer status which most mentors currently hold. In turn, so far as young people only trust mentors because they are not paid to give help, this may threaten the basis for mentoring in its current form. As others (Barry 2000; Philip 2000) have pointed out, there is a tension between the mentor's amateur status as a friend and the status of a professional who has a position of authority over a young person. To be of value, a mentor needs to be seen to be on the young person's side. On the other hand, as noted above, one lesson already learned is that the amateurism of mentor projects (as opposed to mentors) can be a barrier to success, so that professional training of mentor project staff and integration of mentor projects together with other community services are likely to bring advantages.

One way forward on this issue may be to distinguish between mentor projects, which need to be run by professionals, and mentor programmes, which are delivered by amateurs. But, to proceed in this way would be to maintain a distinction which, like the distinction between care and education, may owe more to English history than to the needs of contemporary society. As discussed in chapter 6 of this volume, social pedagogues in Europe are able to represent the interests of children and young people and are accepted by them, while at the same time being valued as professionals by society. It is thus possible to envisage mentors with different levels of professional qualifications, as is the case in other care work professions, as well as a continuing role for community volunteers.

In conclusion, mentoring has already evolved from the original Big Brothers Big Sisters model based solely on befriending between an older person and a younger, less experienced, person. Rather than one model of mentoring, the need over the next few years is to explore alternative ways in which mentor projects can work with volunteers and other community and statutory provisions in order to deliver supports and competencies to at-risk young people. The four defining features of mentors listed above overlap in some degree with the characteristics which define other groups of care workers, while in these other areas, too, there is a growing recognition that care alone is seldom more than a first step towards overcoming problems. If they are to redirect their own lives, at-risk children and young people need more than just care. Recent changes have set the scene for child and adolescent-focused services that offer bridges between care and education, social and health services, and between statutory and voluntary organisations (Department for Education and Skills 2004b; Department of Health 2004). It is likely to take several years for the resulting professions and services to find their final form. Our hope and expectation is that a more developed form of mentoring will have a central part to play in provision for young people who offend or are at risk of offending.

Notes

1   The Youth Justice Board was established by the Home Office under the Crime and Disorder Act 1998, to lead the reforms to the youth justice system. It is a non-departmental public body whose aim is to prevent offending by children and young people.

2   There is a Youth Offending Team (YOT) in every local authority in England and Wales. Each is made up of representatives from the police, probation service, social services, health, education, drugs and alcohol misuse and housing officers. Each YOT has a manager who is responsible for coordinating the work of the youth justice services. YOTs work with children and young people aged 10–17 and their primary aim is to prevent youth crime.

8   Semi-formal care work

The case of private foster care

Edwina Peart, Charlie Owen and
Sofka Barreau

Mrs Arnold is now in her 60s. She has always lived in the same town, on the south coast of England. She lives with her husband, who is retired, but he used to work as an electrician. She started private fostering in 1978. She had four of her own children at the time, aged between 12 and 19, and was missing having young children to look after. One of her friends from the area had been privately fostering children, and told Mrs Arnold about a magazine where parents advertised for foster carers. The parents were mostly Nigerian students, living in London. She got a copy from the newsagents, and through the magazine she contacted a Nigerian couple with a three-week old baby girl. The couple came down the next day and left the baby with her. When the baby was six she went back to live with her parents, but two years later they called to say they had a new baby and would Mrs Arnold look after him, which she did. There was never any shortage of parents wanting a foster carer: Mrs Arnold's name would get passed on, and new families would phone to ask if she could take their baby. Sometimes she could, and sometimes she couldn't. One boy came at a few months old and didn't leave until he was 18. Mrs Arnold thinks his parents went back to Nigeria. She has lost count of the number of children she has fostered over the years. She still has three children with her: their ages are seven, four and a half and eight weeks. The parents all know each other. Mrs Arnold says she does it because she loves children. Her dream is to win the lottery, buy a big house and fill it with children.[1]

The tragic death of Victoria Climbié at the hands of her great aunt and her aunt's boyfriend brought to a wider public attention the fact that a number of children, particularly from West Africa, are sent to Britain for their education (Laming 2003: 3.5). Some live with relatives or someone known to the family, but many live with strangers. In Britain this is known as private fostering. It is also a common practice for Nigerians living in Britain, often as students, to have their young children privately fostered by a British family. This chapter will present a profile of private foster carers drawing on a recent study of private fostering (see Appendix).

Private fostering occurs where a child who is under the age of sixteen is cared for and lives with someone other than their parent or a close relative (or someone with legal parental responsibility) for a period of longer than twenty-eight days.[2] Regulations under the Children Act 1989 state that the local authority should be notified by the carer, and the local authority has a responsibility to look after the general welfare of the child (Department of Health 1991a). Private fostering placements are arranged privately, usually between the parent and the carer, without the involvement of social services. This is similar to the way childminding (or family day care) services are purchased. Under the Children Act 1989, as under previous legislation, childminders are required to register with their local authority, and the local authority in turn has a duty to inspect and approve the arrangement. However, private foster carers are not required to register with the local authority, even though the children in their care are with them for much longer than children are with childminders (Bostock 2003). One recommendation of the Laming inquiry into Victoria Climbié's death was that the government should review the law on the registration of private fostering (Laming 2003: 17.97), although this recommendation was rejected by the government (Department for Education and Skills 2003).

The regulations covering private fostering are, nevertheless, detailed and comprehensive. However, a study by the Social Services Inspectorate in 1994 found that many local authority social services departments did not know about and therefore did not enforce the Children Act regulations concerned with private fostering, and numbers were significantly under reported (Social Services Inspectorate 1994). The Children Act 2004 included measures to strengthen the notification system and establish national minimum standards for private fostering that will be enforced through inspection. The option for a registration system similar to that for childminders may be considered should the guidelines prove insufficient.

As a result of regulations not being enforced, private fostering remains largely hidden from public scrutiny. It is also an area with little research: Bob Holman has called it 'the unknown fostering' (Holman 2002). What research there is points to it predominantly involving families of West African origin (Holman 1973; Philpot 2001), with claims made about the practice being primarily a variant on a cultural practice inappropriately transposed to Britain (Goody 1982). It is also clear that many of the known private fostering arrangements in Britain are transracial placements involving black children being looked after in white families. This may, or may not be significant in understanding the motivations of parents who use this service, or of the carers who supply it. There are also some variations that are less well known about involving children of African Caribbean and Chinese origin being cared for. The Private Fostering study also found that social workers reported an increase in notifications involving teenagers living away from home (Barreau 2004).

Private foster care workers are thus positioned somewhere between an informal carer and a parent, but are also 'workers' in the sense that they are caring for children who are not their own and are, in theory, publicly regulated. They are informal carers in the sense that they are not employed and there are highly variable, if any, arrangements for payment, and they are parents in that they usually have parental experience and care in a domestic setting. They are discussed here as an example of the range of 'care work' that is undertaken in the UK at present. The care offered is the only example of 'childcare' (one word) that takes place away from parental homes. However, the fact that foster care placements are under-reported and under-regulated places these workers in somewhat shady territory, where the care practice is largely invisible to public scrutiny.

The 'Private Fostering' study set out to understand modern day private fostering from the perspectives of all those involved – the carers, the parents and those who had been privately fostered when young[3] (referred to in this chapter as the 'cared for'), including the motivations and experiences of all concerned.[4] However, the public invisibility of private fostering makes it a difficult research topic, as discussed in the project summary in the Appendix.

This chapter will concentrate on those private foster carers who repeatedly foster children, or so called 'traditional' private foster carers. (Those who privately foster teenagers who have left home tend to be very different: they usually only care for one child, who is a friend or relative.) The focus is on the carers, but we will sometimes draw on the interviews with those cared for and parents. The chapter will discuss private fostering as an example of care work that raises many pertinent issues: individual and collective social constructions of care workers and the boundaries between this and parenting; the meeting of different ideologies of parenting and what is considered good practice in both arenas; the monetary encounter and the effect this has on motivations, practice and moral obligations. It is divided into three sections, focusing on: the carers, which includes their motivations, roles and skills; private fostering in practice, which includes how placements begin and end, payment and mistreatment; and race and culture, which includes issues of racism. However, as issues of race and culture pervaded the study, they are inevitably discussed throughout the chapter.

The carers

Care of the young outside the home has always been viewed as women's responsibility, an extension of the mothering role (Cameron et al. 1999). It has traditionally both provided paid employment for women and has also allowed them to pursue employment outside of the home or domestic sphere (Pinchbeck and Hewitt 1973). The long-term care of other people's children is not a new practice, and many references to it can be found in nineteenth-century literature, as outlined in chapter 3. The first legislation to regulate it in Britain was the Infant Life Protection Act 1872. This was introduced as a result of concerns over so-called baby farming, where children could be kept under appalling conditions, often resulting in their deaths (Pinchbeck and Hewitt 1973). The same concerns underlay the first Children Act of 1908. However, the term private fostering does not appear to have been used until the Children Act 1948. All societies, across time, culture and class have experience of women caring for other people's children. Now, as in the past, this is most often met within the family (Reynolds 2001; Wheelock and Jones 2002).

The 29 carers in the Private Fostering study were mainly drawn from those carers who have contact with social services departments and have notified them of the children in their care. These carers were thus used to their practice being scrutinised. Most were married, or had been in the past and had children, including some they had adopted. The children that they privately fostered were mostly of West African origin, with some of Chinese and Caribbean origin. The length of time the foster carers had been fostering ranged from six years to forty-two years, and individual placements from four nights to eighteen years. Carers ranged in age from thirty-four years old to seventy-six years: most were in their late fifties and sixties. They were all white British and the majority lived in the South West of England. All were married, although three had been widowed. In one case a widowed man was interviewed alone, but in all other cases the wife was the main or sole interviewee.

The shortest placements seem to be the result of either placement break-down or a specific request for a specified period. The longest placements are those in which parental contact is severed or care orders sought. Most children are under six months old when placement starts and many return to their parents at around five or six years old.

The intention for a couple to begin private fostering came from the woman in all cases, and some women were fostering alone. Where men took part it was always within marriages and partnerships. It was also essentially an expression of the woman's love of children. However, within this there are various strands. The most common was wanting to continue the paren-tal role or add to the family. For example, one respondent stated: 'We've got two daughters, the oldest one she can't have any children and she always wanted a brother, so that's why.' This continuation of the parental role was clearly an important factor as almost all of the carers we spoke to had children of their own. They tended to start fostering when their birth chil-dren were aged between ten and thirteen. In a few cases carers started when their children were either leaving school, or leaving home. One carer stated that she would have had more children but could not afford to do so.

Approximately a quarter of our sample had previously thought about, or tried, fostering for the local authority. Often they were deterred from this by the expectation (and experience) that children placed by the local authority were 'problem' children. As one carer put it:

> I was going to do fostering with the county [local authority], and we went, my husband and I to the meeting. He gave us the good side of fostering for the county but also the bad side and the bad side, I'm afraid, outweighed the good side. I didn't fancy children peeing up against the bed and I didn't fancy children making fires under the bed and things like that. We discussed it and we decided that we hadn't got a lot, but what we had got we needed to keep. So that put an end to that and we never went back to the county.

Carers were also deterred because they generally wanted to foster babies and the local authorities had to find foster placements for teenagers. As one respondent said:

> I prefer pre-adoption babies under school age, I mean I don't see the point in my fostering children if they're not here, you know what I mean. And I adore babies, always love to have babies and they more or less implied that I was too old for babies and they wanted me to have teenagers. After having six or seven teenagers of my own I wasn't prepared to take on any more so that's when I really went private, so that I could still have the babies.

Another strand within the general motivation of liking children was that of wanting to help people generally. Many carers were proud of the fact that their work enabled parents to pursue careers and education that they would otherwise be excluded from. A few carers detailed specific personal reasons behind their decision to care, such as:

> I have got children of my own but that is why I foster, because I wasn't allowed to keep my children. I was unmarried and young. And so our doctor said he would help me adopt because I couldn't have any more and I said no, I'm not doing that to someone else. So I chose to foster whilst the parents couldn't look after them and yet they didn't lose their kids at the end of the day.

Some carers entered this field through responding to a specific situation where they knew the family and the circumstances. Others did so through personal factors such as the death of a husband, which motivated them to meet their need for communication and love through offering childcare. A final category is that of carers who said they began fostering as this fitted in with their existing childcare responsibilities and their marketable skills.

Interestingly, none of the carers cited money as a motivation. This has also been found with childminders, who rate being at home as more important than the (little) money they get for minding (Mooney et al. 2001). Money was mentioned by some of the cared for, who from their experience felt this could be the only motivation as little care or love was shown. We will return to the theme of payment later in the chapter.

In terms of the entry into private fostering there were two major routes. The first was through advertisements in specialist magazines (e.g. *Nursery World*) and agencies such as the Commonwealth Society. The second was through word of mouth by friends or a family member who was already caring. Those that started through advertisements tended to become established and continue through personal recommendations, as with the earlier portrait of Mrs Arnold. The prohibition of such advertisements was included in the Children Act 1980.

Many of our carers were or had been childminders. Sometimes they were registered, but more often they described providing *ad hoc* care for children in the neighbourhood. This was often encapsulated in statements such as: 'I've always had plenty to do with children, even when I was little. My mum had photographs of me when I was four or five years old with a baby stuck on my hip. My life has always been around children. I can't imagine it without them actually.' None of our carers cited race as a motivating factor for caring. Many of them mentioned being able to care for all children regardless of their race as evidence of the special skills they possessed.

We asked all of our respondents what they felt the role of the carer should be and what skills are required to fulfil this. Almost all described this as a long-term baby-sitting or childminding role, such as these two carers: 'I just took it in my stride, it was just another child that wants a home and love and attention.' 'I thought my role was to help people look after their kids who couldn't obviously look after them at the time.'

Many carers went on to explain that their role was that of a substitute family member. Most often this was defined as a 'grandma' or 'nanny', or sometimes as a substitute parent. The skills required were seen as interchangeable with parenting skills. The fact that care takes place in the care worker's home, and that the provision of a family environment is part of the package means that many carers felt that they cared for their charges in the same ways that they cared for their birth children. Some were referred to as 'mum'. Some carers clearly expressed the opinion that this type of caring allowed them to make their charges their own, including the carer's own culture:

> Well, because you had them from a pup so to speak, from a baby. So therefore you had no worries of being in any sort of bad way. Because at that age, at three months old, you can culture them into your ways. It wasn't as though we were looking after say a ten year old, who could be

a bit more trouble. We had them at three months old so therefore we could nurse them into our way of life.

Another carer explained that:

> I didn't think of it as a role, that had nothing to do with it. The fact was that I loved her, she was mine. I mean I didn't even object to her mother giving birth to her. I accepted that, but it was the fact that she was mine. I'd have laid down my life for her.

This interpretation of caring as 'ownership' of children suggests that rather than a sacrificial 'love' as the primary motivation and reward, this relationship, through its long term and highly committed character, offered intense emotional rewards to foster mothers themselves as well as responsibilities and entitlements. Almost all of the carers stated that the love that they received from the children they cared for was the greatest reward. They also considered that the worst aspect of the job was giving the children up. Whilst some stated clearly that they felt that the child was theirs, for others this did not become apparent until the placement ended and the child left. Interestingly, whilst most carers considered the impact this had upon themselves and their families, only one carer spoke of the impact this separation might have on the child. Speaking of her reasons for giving up private foster caring one carer said:

> I don't like the way the kids are treated really, from pillar to post. I know if a child comes into care sometimes they go from one house to another if they don't get on. But it's for different reasons, I think. These, I know they say they have to go to college, they have to go to work, but they don't really know who they're living with, not when they're bringing them. You know, one visit, it's just not enough. I mean we have lots of nice experiences to remember, but that was our last one and that was a nightmare. I had a nervous breakdown after that. I wouldn't go through that again. And the children, you put the children through too much, seeing them come and go screaming. No, I couldn't go through it again.

This practice questions the boundaries between care work and parenting in that a 'good' carer possesses 'good' parenting skills. This point was agreed by carers, parents and the cared for. Nevertheless, Holman (1973; 2002) found that many of the carers he interviewed would not meet the standards to be accepted as foster carers for local authorities. In the Private Fostering study, some of the carers were local authority foster carers or had been in the past. Similarly, others were or had been registered childminders. However, some certainly would not have met local authority criteria as foster carers, and some should have been excluded even as private foster carers on current regulations.

Whether the carers offer 'good quality' care or not is complicated by the fact that the carer provides care services to a parent usually raised in a very different cultural context. The understandings of the two parties to the agreement, which is usually more implicit than explicit, are imbedded in their individual backgrounds. We will explore this point further through examining the first contact carers have with their charges, the parents and the information that is exchanged. This provides some suggestions as to the position of these workers and the relationships that structure the care experience.

Private fostering in practice

First contact between the carer and the family of the child to be fostered happened in a number of ways, varying from not knowing the parent or the child, to clear arrangements with a known or introduced family for a specified period of time about which everyone was happy and clear. Most carers stated that though they initiated their carer careers in the former way, they maintained them by reputation and word of mouth. In effect, this often meant that many of the children they cared for were related, or at least their parents knew each other.

As already stated, using advertisements to introduce carers was common but could appear insensitive by both parties. But examination contextualises the practice and renders it comprehensible. Advertising gives carers an element of choice, at least in terms of the age and sex of the baby and usually ethnicity also. Some aspects of the care agreement are also in the advertisement in the form of priorities, such as 'no smoking' and 'no animals'. The Private Fostering study did not ask specific questions about how carers distinguished between advertisements, but did ask about circumstances where carers would refuse a child. Carers initially stated that they accept all children, but closer examination showed that factors such as the length of placement, how clean the child appears, how healthy it is, how happy it is, and whether or not it has special needs were all considered and influenced the decision reached. In contrast to the 'ownership' approach noted above, some carers stated that they insisted the parents visit and loved the child as a condition of caring, as illustrated by this carer:

> Oh yes, I insist on that, they've got to have close contact because they've got to know who they belong to, where they come from. So I like them to visit at least once a fortnight and when they're younger they get used to it, you know, they do know that's mummy and daddy and I have photos of mummy and daddy around the house and we show, that's mummy and that's daddy. When they phone up and they talk to the children, she talks to mum, she comes over is that my mummy on the phone, I say yes … and she says 'hello mummy' and that and she talks to mummy. I like

them to have a close contact with their parents, so that they know, and
I like them to go home regular even if it's only for a weekend.

Many carers met and were left with the child at the same time. This was
usually preceded by a telephone conversation in which both parties gathered
information. The placing of children in this way is an element of the practice
that was presented as cold and uncaring on the part of parents, often by the
carers themselves. However, many carers also reported that they had met
couples who made arrangements to start care at a later date and who failed
to return with the child or provide any explanation. Carers seemed to view
this element of the practice in two ways. Firstly, some considered that their
reputation was such that the parents were reassured before meeting them
and that the meeting itself was something of a formality. The second view
was that the birth parents, due in large part to their culture, were unable to
appreciate the skills required for good parenting, as evidenced by their casual
delegation of the care of their child. Carers also complained that parents
sometimes returned for the child after a few days or weeks and terminated
care – giving reasons such as the carer being too old. Analysis of the initial
contact between the carer and the parent provides insights into how vulnerable the situation is for all of the parties involved including the foster carer.

Remuneration was another area in which the boundaries between care
work and parenting, volunteering and working were blurred. The situation
was very diverse. Payment ranged from £10 per week to £300 per month.
This range was still well below what the Fostering Network considers to be
the minimum necessary to cover the costs of fostering a child, without any
element of reward for the carer. In 2003, their recommended allowance
ranged between £106 and £222 per week depending on the age of the child
(Fostering Network 2005). Some Private Fostering study carers were paid a
small amount of money but the parent provided clothes, paid for treats,
some food and anything the child needed. In some instances carers had been
assisted by social services departments when parents failed to pay. However,
the childcare offered was always cheap. Money was clearly not a motivating
factor, but neither was it a prohibiting factor. Only a few carers felt that the
money they received covered their costs. One carer explained that: 'When
I had Gary I used to get ten pounds a week, because I knew his mum couldn't
afford much. But then I was able to get his family allowance, it just about
covers costs.'

Where costs were not met this could be for a variety of reasons. These
included the particular eating habits of a child, birthday and Christmas
presents, incidental expenses such as presents for birthday parties that carers
had to meet.

Some carers complained that parents exploit them, such as this one:

Her mother was awful. When I said to her, 'you know, well you've got to
pay for her keep, he's a pensioner, I don't go to work, where do you

think the money comes from?' Well, she said, 'I look on you as my mother'. I said well, 'don't look on me as your mother'. I said 'I've got enough children I don't need you'. I said 'if you don't want to pay for her then you just have to take her back'.

This carer felt that the parents expected her to subsidise the childcare costs in her role as surrogate grandmother. Most carers stated that if the money stopped they would continue caring for the child they had become attached to. This was not just a theoretical question as many of the carers in this study found themselves in this position and they continued to care. One carer who had received no payments for a year explained: 'It's not his fault, he's still got to be fed and clothed. But as I say his daddy had got kidney failure and he's on income support so you know. If you love children you can't do it.'

None of our sample said they would stop caring if payment ceased. Some stated that they would seek advice and others that essentially nothing would change. This is evidence of their commitment to those they cared for and the fact that they saw them as part of their family. The carers repeatedly emphasised that what you needed to be a good foster carer was love for the children: some were critical of foster carers who worked for social services, because those carers were doing it for money: 'It's not done for the love of kids, it's done for bloody money and I'm against that sort of thing . . . You know what I mean. I don't think nobody should foster not for that, not for money. It's not about money: it's about a kid's life.'

Two other factors relating to finance need to be mentioned. One carer spoke of the impact on the household budget that assistance from social services made when payment from a parent stopped. This clearly showed that though the amounts received from parents were small, they had a significant impact on the total household budget and the family's earning potential. Some carers also stated that they would have had more children themselves if they had greater financial resources. Private fostering can thus also be a way of raising a child as your own with subsidy from its parents.

Private fostering has been highlighted as an especially vulnerable status for children (e.g. Utting 1997). The private nature of the arrangement can mean there is no one protecting the child's interests and that there is little redress if mistreatment is identified. This special vulnerability was confirmed by the Private Fostering study.

Issues of mistreatment by private foster carers and allegations of mistreatment were explored in interviews with those who had previously been cared for, parents and carers. Among carers, three said that they had been accused of abusing a child. In two cases this concerned physical abuse and in one sexual abuse. In no instance were the accusations upheld or charges made. However, data from those cared for and parents show that carers often fail to protect their charges and sometimes both they and their families actively perpetrate cruelty against the children in their care. Four of those cared for in private foster care (out of 12) revealed incidents of abuse. One said they had been physically abused, one that they had been sexually abused, a third reported mental and physical abuse and a fourth said they had been both sexually and mentally abused. This evidence questions the skills and competencies of carers and is a major criticism of private fostering, particularly that which takes place outside public scrutiny.

Culture and race

As we have already noted, the carers and the parents mostly had different ethnic and cultural backgrounds. Carers held ambivalent opinions about the culture and practices of the parents whose children they cared for, as can be seen in the following statements:

> They've got a different culture to us, different altogether and I say I've only understood since I was doing the private fostering. Most of them don't bring up their own children, but they always provide for their elders. You know, so I am taking the place of the grandma more or less because the grandmas are out there and they're here.
>
> Well it's their culture so you don't feel anything about them. It's just their way of life. You can't condemn someone else's culture, can you? That's the way I see it anyway. I mean if my daughter said to me she was going to put her children into care then I would think twice about that because it's not her culture, and I wouldn't like it one little bit. But with these it's just their culture and there's not much you can do about that.

Most carers stated that it is important for the children in their care to be familiar with their own culture. They also detailed the ways in which they were able to support this in terms of hair and skin care and sometimes food. This level of skill could be related to the fact that most carers in this study had access to social work support in the form of group meetings and discussions about culture and caring. Nevertheless, the carers had distinct criticisms of what were viewed as cultural practices. Carers viewed the maintenance of the culture of the cared for as important whilst simultaneously regarding it as 'backward' and inferior to British culture. Carers repeatedly pointed out the potential benefits of being cared for in a white environment. They thought that – somehow – knowing two cultures intimately would present the young people with an avenue of escape from racism. Some carers felt that an adequate cultural input could be gained from regular parental visits alone and required no specific action on their part.

The most positive statements seemed to come from carers recalling their inclusion in cultural celebrations and being made to feel very welcome and special, as the following carer vividly recounted:

I mean when we go up there, for instance we went up there one time and they had a party or a celebration of someone that just had a baby. There were maybe about fifty or sixty people, all coloured, all in the house and we're the only two white people. And the time we left I think everybody shook our hand. 'Oh you're the foster people of our friend, oh glad to meet you'. And well we were so overwhelmed, we were welcomed there, it was unbelievable.

In addition to questions about the importance of culture, experiences of racism, both personal and in relation to their charges were discussed in interviews. Carers were much better able to identify racism directed against themselves than against the young people. One carer reported direct racially motivated comments from her local community, such as: 'When I first started I had people used to take me and say, "what you been down the coal hole?" '

During interviews carers were often hesitant and unsure whether or not to label behaviour directed against their charges in school or in the wider community as racist. Some carers felt that for various reasons such as age, temperament and locality the children they cared for had escaped racism. For example, one carer said:

We was here probably about six months when we had the last black children, but no one round here seemed to worry because you know they were so well behaved, they were only young. I mean afterwards they were so well behaved you know everybody said what marvellous kids they were. They weren't bullied at all at school, they mixed well at school.

However, some carers reported that racism directed at the children they cared for had had a significant impact on their family lives, such as this carer, who stated:

The police had to move us. We had a terrible time for two years over Tony. It was fine until he reached the age of six and he wanted to go out and play, but they wouldn't have it. They would not let him go out and play. He went to school, they followed him down the school, it was terrible. We had to fill in a form anytime anything happened. In the end it got so bad the police moved us.

Most carers who identified racism did so in relation to the school and most were satisfied with the ways in which the issue was dealt with. Only one carer felt that the school did not support her fostered child. Moreover, only one carer acknowledged racism within her own family. By contrast, all of those cared for raised such issues. A comparison of attitudes to racism between the carers and those who had been privately fostered (the 'cared for') showed that carers were, for the most part, unable to give the support those cared for felt they needed. From the perspective of the cared for, school was a site of regular racist incidents which were rarely adequately dealt with. The cared for also recounted racist attitudes held by carers and their families and displayed towards them.

Carer attitudes to race and culture can also be gleaned from the carers' reports of relationships with parents. Some carers were interested in the parents they worked for and held positive views of them. This was usually based on criteria such as providing well for their family, being ambitious and studying and working hard, dispensing generous gifts to the carer and including them in parties and celebrations. As one carer said:

> The little one, her mum is at university, she's studying to be a nurse. As well as studying, they go to work as well these Nigerians, they're really hard working the women, they put their self through it all. She says, 'I could never manage to do it without your help'. She makes beautiful yellow rice and it's all got peppers in it, and when she comes down to visit she brings a big carton. And she'll bring down lots of chicken cooked for us, that's presents for us you know.

However, some carers held a disapproving view of the birth parents. This was often based on feeling that they, as carers, were being exploited both financially and emotionally. Sometimes this was related to payment, but also to the bonds the carer had developed with the child. Many carers felt this placed them in a vulnerable position and that parents used this to assert their power. One carer speaking of a parent said:

> She complained because he wouldn't call her 'mum' and things like that you know. And then things just went from bad to worse. She brought me two children, she asked me if I would look after these two children and I said 'no I really didn't want to take on anymore'. Every time I said 'no' to something, she said, 'oh I'll put Peter somewhere else then. I'll take him somewhere else', you know. So every time we said 'yes'.

In addition to feeling exploited and explicitly criticising parents, carers often implied that many of the parents they had contact with, including the ones they had respect for, were somewhat incompetent. This was often directly in relation to a specific element of childcare. One carer typically stated:

> When he first came he couldn't chew, he didn't know how to chew. I can remember the night he came. I thought well, he's twenty-two months, we had fish and chips and I got him sausage and chips. I cut up his sausage and I sat him at the table. And he just sat there. Anyway I put a piece in his mouth and it just stayed in his mouth. Then I got him a packet of crisps, I tell you he didn't even know how to put his hand in

this packet of crisps and take out a crisp, I had to show him. We had to go like this, make out we was chewing. It took a little while, but then he used to hold it all in his mouth. He used to put a spoon in and you'd think he's eating. But he wasn't, it was like a hamster in his mouth. And then they brought a bottle down with him, and I didn't realise it was in the pocket of the case. I got it out, thought what's that in there and it was a bottle and the top of it was cut off. So they must have been feeding him, with whatever they give, through the bottle and that's why he didn't know how to chew.

This extract shows that the cultural context of the parental home was completely overlooked. The carer did not consider the cultural specificity of the food she was offering, or the use of utensils. The parents were judged from a white, British standpoint and found lacking.

For some carers their negative attitudes to parents were directed at individuals. Even within families carers could commend the mother and state that the father was useless. For others, criticisms tended to be directed at 'them', against cultural or racial groupings.

A common theme of carer criticism was that many birth parents expected their children to display independence and competence in caring for themselves from an early age. One carer expressed extreme disapproval of such practice: 'Their mother was, and still is – can I say it – a bitch. She's never been a mother to them. Even when they went home from here. I think before she was ten, she went to night work and left those two kids on their own.'

Carers frequently referred to this type of negligence, which was viewed as a culturally accepted practice by parents. Carers also held similarly disparaging beliefs relating to the way parents disciplined their children and their expectations of responsibility for chores. These factors were also mentioned by the cared for.

A third area in which carer criticism was high is that of contact. Carers reproached parents for lack of contact, inconsistent contact and for holding unrealistic expectations of attachment with their child when they visited. Many carers described having to provide support to the mothers when the children were visiting home, as they had no knowledge of their routines, or a sufficient attachment to them. All carers spoke of the ease with which the children settled back into the carer's home after a visit to the parental home. Many carers also stated that their charges were reluctant and apprehensive when required to visit the parental home. One carer revealed some of the tensions inherent in private fostering when she said:

When you foster care you take a lot of their security off them [the children]. They're so unsure they never know how long they're gonna be there, whether they're going to be wanted, what will happen to them. It's terrible, it's wicked actually you know. The parents don't realise how much cruelty they're inflicting on their children you know. The cruelty is in the mind of the child, you know. They just push them through the door, 'bye see you in a fortnight'. It's like leaving a parcel and hoping it'll get delivered to the person it's meant for. It's all wrong.

The role of the carer and her relationship with the children she cared for is positioned within two distinct cultural settings. It is outside of the scope of this chapter and its focus to delve into West African culture. However, several observations can be made. There is clearly some convergence between the two cultural expressions of care work that allow parents to use and carers to offer the service. Both parties agree that in practice it resembles extended family care. It is at this point that understandings seem to diverge. It may be that parenthood in a West African context places less emphasis than in the UK on the affectional bond between mother and child. Within West African culture, caring for the child is not the exclusive role of the biological parent, but can be and is shared within the wider community (Goody and Groothues 1979).

In the United Kingdom, on the other hand, 'good' parenting is commonly understood to include a primary attachment to the mother. This is considered to be particularly important in early infancy. Carers thus feel that by providing a secure attachment they offer, in effect, better parenting. However, shared childcare within the community in many black and West African communities does not dispute or undermine parenthood. It supports parents and recognises their many roles and the component tasks of child rearing (Barrow 1996; Goody and Groothues 1979). Grandmothers and others can legitimately mother children, and this is not seen as contesting the parenting skills of the biological parents. Private fostering across cultures can leave the carers and the parents conceiving of the practice in different ways.

Conclusion

Private foster carers provide childcare services in a manner that essentially allows them to continue their parenting role. This intimate and frequently long-term commitment is clearly rewarding. Many of them speak of the day-to-day freedom that they enjoy in relation to their charges and the instinctual nature of their care. In some ways they perceive themselves as selling a service, in others ways they reject this notion and point out the similarity between the care they offer and the way they raised their birth children.

Their implicit claim to the moral high ground in childcare, based largely on their low rates of pay in comparison to local authority foster carers, is not justified by the evidence. They make choices about the children they care for. It is also unclear what proportion of them would be accepted as local authority carers. The regulations governing private fostering are fairly stringent, but they are rarely enforced, so carers operate largely outside a regulatory framework. This is particularly the case for carers who are not known to the local authority, but also even for those who are. Two of the carers we interviewed have birth children who were placed in local authority care. The private fostering regulations state that this situation provides grounds for refusing to allow a carer to offer childcare, but this had not been acted upon.

In terms of the level of skills that carers possess, there are several areas where guidance and training would clearly be helpful. All of the carers interviewed in this study spoke of the difficulties they experienced when a placement ends. Training could help to prepare them for this. All of the carers expressed appreciation for group training sessions in which they had participated in the past, but which were no longer available, that had provided them with training in hair and skin care and insights into culture.

The transracial nature of the placements presents many deeply worrying issues. From the carers' perspective, there is an implicit assumption that they provide care that is at minimum just as good as that of the parental offer and more often a lot better. There are many, sometimes veiled, criticisms in their descriptions of the parents that they have contact with. This is often specifically directed at their parenting skills and differences in cultural mores pertaining to childcare. Carers also claim a greater general and individual knowledge of children.

For carers, issues of race and culture are almost overlooked with regard to the children they care for. They are more often present, though, in relation to the child's parents. Carers seem unaware of the possible impact of this on the child who needs to love and be loved by its birth parents and to develop a positive image of themselves and their place within their ethnic group.

Carers recognise in part the barriers they are breaking down for the children they care for in terms of language and culture. They are less able to see the mediating influence of racism. This difference is significant and it relates to the relative power and position in society of white working-class carers and the black, minority ethnic parents they work for. All parties are vulnerable.

There are three factors that are likely to influence the future of private fostering as described here. First, current government attention means it is unlikely that the practice will continue in such an unregulated way (Department for Education and Skills 2005). At present private fostering stands as a glaring anomaly in childcare, where other services are not delivered in this way. Second, the cohort of carers interviewed in the Private Fostering study were generally at the end of their working lives. Many stated that the children currently cared for would be their last placement. Some had already ceased their carer careers. It is also worth repeating that for most of our carers motherhood provided their defining role, in the sense that they did not participate in paid work outside of the home whilst raising their children. This traditional role is no longer the norm. Most mothers now work alongside raising children (Wheelock and Jones 2002), and have fewer children. Third, evidence from the cared for and from parents suggests that this type of fostering is no longer widespread and is being replaced by private fostering within the parents' community of origin. Together, these factors would seem to undermine the continuation or growth of the form of private fostering described here. That said, as other forms of semi-formal foster care provision develop, such as kinship care for looked-after children, issues raised in this chapter – for example, about training and payment – will have wider relevance for the future of care work.

Notes

1   This is a composite portrait, based on a number of interviews. A pseudonym has been used.
2   The official definition includes children who are cared for outside of their home but where their parents may not be involved in making the arrangement. This would include young students in language schools, sports trainees, unaccompanied young immigrants and asylum seekers and young people who leave home. However, our research concentrates on a particular group, those who use private fostering as a form of childcare.
3   The project did not interview children and young people who were currently being privately fostered.
4   The research project was funded by the Department of Health. However, the Department is not responsible for the interpretations and views expressed here.

9 Informal care across the generations

Ann Mooney and June Statham

Jane[1] and her husband Robert are both 54 and have two children. Their son and his wife have just had their first child and their daughter, a single parent, has a three and a half year old. Jane is one of nine children. Her father is 91 and has recently moved to live with one of Jane's sisters, and her in-laws are in their seventies. There are many examples of informal care in Jane's life. She and her sisters helped their parents and subsequently their father when their mother died. When her daughter's marriage broke up, Jane found herself supporting her daughter as well as helping her sister care for their father. The stress of supporting her family led to her own ill health and she resigned from her job as a learning support assistant. Although this had a detrimental effect on her pension, she felt she was unable to continue with both her work and her caring responsibilities. Jane now works 10 hours a week as a supervisor in an out-of-school club, which gives her much satisfaction, though she foresees having to give this up as her caring responsibilities increase. Her sister is finding care of their father difficult and Jane provides respite care. Her brothers are largely exempted from this because, according to Jane, they are the main breadwinners in their families. Jane provides emotional and practical support to her in-laws and to her son and daughter. She has her granddaughter to stay at least once a week, but does not want to provide regular childcare while her children work, though is happy to help in an emergency. She 'keeps an eye' on an elderly neighbour and helps him as and when she can. Jane sees caring as being what families are about, 'you get back what you give', but says it is also in her nature to care.

This thumbnail sketch of an informal carer, taken from a recent study exploring work and caring responsibilities among people in their 50s and

60s (Mooney et al. 2002), illustrates what informal care across the generations can look like. Jane's story shows us that informal care is complex and diverse. It is not a static entity and, as we shall see, does not necessarily have a clear beginning and end. We see one impact of caring – withdrawal from the labour market – and we note a reluctance to take on regular childcare. This scenario also raises a number of questions. What defines informal care? How extensive is it, and is demand waxing or waning? What are the characteristics of informal carers, and what impact does caring have on carers' lives? This chapter explores these questions by drawing on the data from two recent studies: the 'Fifty Plus' study referred to above (Mooney et al. 2002), and the 'Four Generation' study which looked at work and care across and within 12 four-generation families (Brannen et al. 2004). The chapter concludes by considering the future for this type of care and its relationship to formal services.

Defining informal care

When people talk about informal care, they tend to think of care provided within the family, for example for grandchildren while their parents work or study, or for elderly parents as they become less able to manage without help. Indeed, the majority of informal care *is* provided for parents and parents-in-law (Evandrou 1995), and relatives are still the largest providers of childcare in England (e.g. Woodland et al. 2002). Yet, informal care embraces much more than childcare and eldercare. It includes care for a child, partner or other relative with a disability or chronic illness, and care provided to friends or neighbours who are sick or elderly. Parents sharing the school run, having children back for tea and helping out in emergencies are all forms of informal care that are often overlooked, despite their importance for those parents who rely on them to fill the gaps in their childcare arrangements. Finally, the care that fathers and step-fathers provide while mothers work is a form of informal care that has been included in some studies (e.g. Woodland et al. 2002) and excluded from others (e.g. Wheelock and Jones 2002). In this chapter, we focus particularly on informal childcare provided by grandparents, and informal eldercare.

The commitment based on friendship or relationship, which underlies informal caring activity, distinguishes it from much of the care work described elsewhere in this book. But it has other defining features. Informal care is marked by being largely unpaid, at least in financial terms, a point we return to later in the chapter. It does not require particular qualifications or training, is unregulated and usually home-based. Frequency and duration may also affect what is counted informal care by researchers. In the Fifty Plus study, informal care was defined as care provided at least once a month for kin, friends or neighbours because they are ill, frail or have a disability, or for grandchildren because their parents are working or studying. Other studies have restricted their sample to those providing significant amounts of care, for example 20 hours a week or more.

Furthermore, how informal care itself is defined is important. All too often, care is thought of in terms of the physical tasks involved with personal care, with less credence given to other practical and emotional support. In the Fifty Plus study, eldercare was broadly defined to include personal care, domestic tasks such as cleaning and shopping, providing transport and managing finances, although emotional support was excluded. Other studies have adopted an even broader definition, describing caring activities as 'the important dimensions of day-to-day activities which are so central to the sustaining of family lives and personal relationships – helping, tending, looking out for, thinking about, talking, sharing, and offering a shoulder to cry on' (Williams 2004: 17).

A further dimension is that the definitions adopted by researchers may not reflect the 'lived experience' of those providing informal care. People often do not regard themselves as carers of an older relative, for example, until they are undertaking considerable amounts of care, particularly personal care. A 57-year-old teacher who had been caring for her father for many years illustrated this in the Fifty Plus study, when she said:

> I mean I filled in your form and acknowledged I was a carer, but somehow in there 'I'm going to do my dad' isn't quite the same as saying 'I'm my father's carer' ... certainly not until I got involved with outside agencies who kept telling me I was a carer, but up to that point I don't think I saw myself in that role.

Likewise, care of grandchildren does not necessarily evoke images of a carer in the mind of a grandparent. The same interviewee went on to explain that looking after her grandchildren did not make her think 'I'm assisting my daughter or that I'm a carer, I just think I'm having the boys for the night. It's all of those things that you write down as family.'

The extent of informal care

National surveys demonstrate the important role that informal care plays in meeting the social care needs of individuals. Nearly seven million adults in five million households in Great Britain were providing care for sick, disabled or elderly relatives and friends in 2000 (Maher and Green 2002). Estimates of the economic value of this care range from almost £14 billion to £57 billion, the equivalent of a second NHS budget (Carers UK 2002). These figures do not include care of non-disabled children or grandchildren, although such childcare is another significant type of informal care. In a large-scale survey of English parents about their childcare arrangements and preferences, nearly three-quarters reported using family and friends to provide childcare in the previous year compared with just over half who had used formal provision (Woodland et al. 2002). Some parents had used both types of care, but only one in eight relied solely on formal childcare arrangements. Other research has shown how parents using formal care often also rely on informal arrangements, for example to take or collect children or ferry them between settings (Skinner 2003; Wheelock and Jones 2002).

Our own studies revealed how informal care is fluid in terms of duration and amounts of care. Among the older workers and recent retirees surveyed for the Fifty Plus study, almost half (48 per cent) were informal carers or had been so in the previous 12 months. People moved in and out of caring roles for different family members over time, as well as responding to changes in the type and amount of care needed. A significant number of carers (41 per cent) thought their care responsibilities would increase in the future, and over half who were not currently caring thought they might need to do so in the following five years.

Among people in their fifties and sixties, providing eldercare may be more common than childcare for grandchildren. The most common recipients of informal care in the Fifty Plus study were elderly parents and, in particular, mothers and fathers rather than in-laws. One in five were supporting both elderly relatives *and* caring for grandchildren (Table 9.1).

Kinship hierarchies still influence the care of relatives, with help being sought first from a spouse or partner, followed by another relative living in the same household, a daughter, daughter-in-law, son, other relatives, then friends and neighbours (Carers UK 2001). However, the Fifty Plus study found that while it was more common for both men and women to provide care for their own parent than for their parent-in-law, the difference

Table 9.1 Carers by gender and who they care for

	Female carers (n = 374) %	Male carers (n = 108) %	All carers (n = 482) %
Caring for:			
Parent	48	37	45
Parent-in-law	18	29	20
Grandchild (maternal)	26	19	25
Grandchild (paternal)	16	9	15
Friend/neighbour	13	16	14
Spouse/partner	7	8	7
Aunt/aunt-in-law	8	5	7
Son/daughter (ill/ disabled)	4	4	4
Other	5	5	5

Source: Fifty Plus study

Note: Columns total more than 100% as carers could be providing multiple care.

was especially marked for women. Nearly three times as many women cared for their own parent as for a parent-in-law, whereas men were almost as likely to say they provided care for a parent-in-law as for their own mother or father (Table 9.1). One explanation for this, and one that was borne out by interviews with carers in the Fifty Plus study, is that an important aspect of men's caring role lies in assisting their wife or partner with the support of her parents, rather than taking on a primary care role themselves.

Gender differences are also apparent in the number of hours spent in caregiving. Although the same study found that almost as many men as women provided care, women did more of it. Women were also more likely to be the main carer and to provide personal and domestic care while men were much more likely to say they helped with managing finances. There was little evidence that informal care was restricted to particular groups of employees. Caregiving activities were undertaken by men and women, working full-time and part-time, and at all levels of the organisation. The main difference was that women's caregiving tended to be more extensive, and that working full time or being in a household where both partners worked, appeared to limit the hours of care that could be provided.

Why do people care?

Both the Fifty Plus and the Four Generation studies provide information on the factors that come into play when people make decisions about taking on informal care for relatives, friends or neighbours. Such factors include an individual's availability to care, which may be limited by employment, distance, ill-health or other responsibilities; family patterns of reciprocity and autonomy; norms and preferences for types of care; and the availability of alternative formal services. The decisions that people make in such circumstances often reflect a strong sense of moral commitment and a concern to 'do the right thing' in their particular situation (Williams 2004).

Availability and willingness to provide informal care

Most carers are of working age and in Britain some 13 per cent of full-time employees and 17 per cent of part-time employees combine work and care (Maher and Green 2002). Yet there is considerable evidence that carers can experience substantial difficulties in combining care and employment, especially as hours of care increase (Evandrou 2003; Speiss and Schneider 2003). Rising employment among women in their fifties, who in the past have traditionally been the main providers of informal care, may affect the continuing availability of this source of care. For example grandparents, particularly those in their fifties, may not be available to care for grandchildren because of their own work commitments. Nor are they necessarily willing to stop work in order to become available. The carers interviewed in the Fifty Plus study often enjoyed their paid work and were very committed to it. The identity they achieved through paid work seemed particularly important to women of this generation, who had often withdrawn from full-time employment for childrearing. Not only did they enjoy their work, but it provided them with another identity and brought a greater sense of self esteem. Typical was a clerical worker, who said that 'I've spent so much of my sort of early married life [being] somebody's wife, somebody's mum, and that's a part of coming out to work that I'm me . . . I do like coming out to work.'

Financial reasons also played a part in respondents' decisions about taking on caring roles, especially for women in the 'fifty plus' generation who often had insufficient pension contributions to enable them to leave work or reduce their hours in order to provide informal care. Women in this generation were unlikely to have had continuous employment careers. Although not always withdrawing entirely from paid work, the jobs they took while their children were young had been those that could be fitted around care of their children. These jobs were usually part time and short term. Since returning to the labour market, often developing new careers, many of these women were keen to continue working so that they could maximise their pension contributions.

Employment considerations were not the only reason why some people were not in a situation where they were able – or willing – to take on a caring role. The most common reason given for not providing care in the Fifty Plus survey (apart from not knowing anyone who needed it) was that the respondent lived too far away from the person needing care. It is well established that proximity can determine the extent and nature of participation in eldercare (Joseph and Hallman 1998). Geographical proximity not only affects which kin become informal carers, but also the ability of other family members to support the carer. A father in the Fifty Plus study, whose daughter had a severe learning disability, had considered getting a job nearer his family because 'they [wider family] are all living in [another part of the country] and it's just that much too far'. In the Four Generation study, all the households in half the families had continued to live close to one another, while in the remaining families, at least one household in each family was living at a significant distance from the others. Proximity was a key factor in the ability to provide care, particularly regular childcare.

Some carers were prepared to take on a certain amount of informal care, but drew limits around this. We saw in our thumbnail sketch at the start of this chapter that Jane did not want to provide regular childcare for her grandchildren while their parents worked, and she was not alone in this choice. In both the Fifty Plus and Four Generation studies, grandparents expressed reluctance to take on significant amounts of childcare. Those grandparents who did provide full-time childcare (or had done so in the past), such as a 63-year-old paternal grandmother who stopped working to care full time for her first grandchild, were rare. Rather, those providing childcare tended to do it on a part-time basis or as a back-up in an emergency.

If they were working, they fitted childcare in around other work, such as the full-time care assistant who worked atypical hours and cared for her grandson one day a week on her day off. This reflects findings from the 1999 British Social Attitudes Survey, which showed that grandmothers were more likely to provide childcare when their daughters (or daughters-in-law) worked part time, and were often reluctant to take on a more substantial caring role (Dench and Ogg 2002).

The primary reason for this reluctance appeared to be the restrictions that such a commitment would place on grandparents in terms of their own lives. A grandfather[2] in the Four Generation study, the only one of his generation among the study families to provide childcare, had reduced his working hours to pursue other interests in his life. He was clear that he would not want to care for his two young grandsons on a full-time basis: 'Five whole days a week, every week? I think that would not be reasonable . . . I am happy to be a part-time grandparent . . . I'm getting all excited about the fact that I do one afternoon from one 'til seven, once a week, sometimes only once every 10 days.'

Comments from interviewees in the Four Generation study, when they were asked to select an 'ideal' childcare arrangement for a seven-month-old child whose parents were working, also reflected a perception that full-time childcare might be too much of an imposition on grandparents. A full-time working mother, whose sister looked after her children, described the ideal for the seven-month-old as a childminder because it provided one-to-one attention unlike a nursery, but rejected the grandparent care option because they have 'other things they want to do, you'd be tying them down'. A grandmother, who did not work but cared for her grandchildren frequently on a part-time basis, chose as her ideal scenario a combination of grandparent and nursery care, saying that being with grandparents full time would 'completely take their [grandparents] life away'.

Other reasons for grandparents not providing childcare included the fear that 'it would spoil the relationship within the family' and that being the main carer could mean that visiting grandparents was no longer seen as a 'special' time. But even with this reluctance to take on substantial childcare, sometimes for very practical reasons, family obligations could remain strong as shown by this grandfather in the Four Generation study who said if his son and daughter-in-law were to ask for help with childcare 'I morally *would* say yes. I *know* from experience that after a couple of days [of the grandchildren], we're dead. They wear us out . . . But I couldn't say no.'

Reciprocity and family obligations

A sense of commitment and duty towards family members underpinned many decisions to provide informal care. Reciprocity or repaying parents for earlier help was a recurrent motivational theme in both studies. A female carer in the Fifty Plus study explained that she felt there was no choice (about caring) 'because look what our parents do for us when we're young, and that's the time to pay it back isn't it?' Emotional ties and kinship obligations influenced this reciprocity, as in the case of this mother from the Four Generations study: 'Well, I'd hope that they [sons] would be brought up in the way that they would – I mean, my nan's cared for us in her time. We're now caring for her, the same as I will care for my parents when they . . .'.

Intergenerational relations that led family members to provide support to one another across the generations in this way characterised some families labelled as 'solidaristic' in the Four Generation study. Just as the older generations had been given help with childcare by their mothers, so they in turn wanted to help their children and grandchildren. Such help was then 'repaid' when elderly parents needed support, as this grandmother explained: 'My mum and dad need me, and I am their carer now . . . I really felt that my mum had given me so much when I was young and needed a lot of help.'

Such reciprocity can extend beyond immediate family members to providing informal care for neighbours or friends, as illustrated by two female carers in the Fifty Plus study. A 58-year-old, employed full time as a care assistant working atypical hours, provided much support for her 81-year-old neighbour who had helped her when she had a young family: 'Her and her husband – ever since we've moved in here, have always been very good to us, you know. And to me it's no hardship.' And a 56-year-old carer who worked part time as a classroom assistant described how her 81-year-old friend, who had no family living close to her, had become increasingly dependent upon her. When asked why she cared for this friend she explained how, when she started working in school, her friend, an experienced teacher, had taken her under her wing: 'she was very kind to me. I was very green . . . very apprehensive about everything, and she was like another mum. She looked after me for years.'

These accounts might suggest that the giving of care is made in some calculated way with the expectation that there will be a return. This seemed not to be the case. In explanations of the care between kin, interviewees from both studies talked in terms of love and caring relationships. A daughter talking about helping her parents said, 'You do it because you love them don't you?'; and a great-grandmother, explaining why when she was young and with young children of her own she cared for her grandmother, explained that 'It all boils down to love doesn't it? . . . She loved us, so we loved her in return.'

Norms and preferences for type of care

We have seen how help with childcare was repeated across generations in some families with reciprocity a strong motivational factor. Another reason for keeping childcare within the family is the belief that care by relatives, followed by friends, is the next best thing to parental care. Several studies report that in choosing childcare parents say that being able to trust the carer is of most importance in their choice (e.g. Mooney et al. 2001; Woodland et al. 2002). Trust is a critical component in the relationship between parent and childcarer since parents need to know and trust that in their absence their child will be well cared for. Previous knowledge of the carer encourages such trust and this is further reinforced if there are biological ties. Large-scale survey data of parents shows that in choosing grandparents for childcare, the most frequently mentioned reason is trust, followed by the grandparents' affection for the child, and the way they look after children in the same way as parents (Henthorne and Harkins 2004; Woodland et al. 2002).

Cost, on the other hand, seems to be less of a reason for choosing informal care. Only one in seven of all informal providers in a national survey of childcare was chosen for this reason, although few households relying on informal arrangements paid for childcare (Woodland et al. 2002). In fact, grandparents seem particularly reluctant to accept monetary reward from their children in payment for childcare (Mooney et al. 2002; Wheelock and Jones 2002), although they often receive payment in kind in the form of a gift or treat (Woodland et al. 2002). We have also seen how help with childcare can be repaid at a much later stage when adult children provide help to elderly parents.

Responses to the hypothetical childcare scenario presented in the Four Generation study suggested that a key reason why grandparents were often selected as the best childcare option was because they were family and could therefore be trusted. Furthermore, grandparents were seen to have a special, close relationship to the child and often shared the same values as parents, a view expressed below by a great-grandmother, grandfather and mother:

> Well I think, if the grandparents could do it, I think; because it's blood relations. And I think they'd care more . . . I think the grandparents, if they'd be willing to do it. I'd feel more safe and relaxed, than having a nursery or a childminder.

> There's an inner feeling, connection, between family than you would have between the childminder and the nursery . . . The influence of that person may be completely alien to *you*, or your family set-up . . . So I would think grandparents are more inclined to be in sympathy with the way the child is being brought up.

> I think their [children] main learning comes out of being with a one-to-one adult . . . they need that bond . . . [Grandparents] have an invested emotional interest in the welfare of the child . . . to leave them with their grandparents is the next best thing to us . . . it's their flesh and blood.

Looking at the responses of women only, grandparents (either alone or in combination with another type of care) were the most frequent choice in response to the scenario, though more so among great-grandmothers and less so among their granddaughters. Among grandmothers and their daughters, however, the majority chose formal care, though often in combination with grandparent care because, as we have seen, of the restrictions that full-time childcare could place upon grandparents. But in reality, formal services figured far less than in this hypothetical situation. Across all three generations in each of the 12 families that participated in the Four Generation study, very little formal childcare had been used, either currently or in the past. More of the parent generation had used non-parental care than was the case in previous generations, but even so, formal care had been used by only four families (a nursery, an au pair and, in two families, a childminder). And in none of these cases had there been sole use of formal care throughout the period it was needed: informal care (by the child's father or a grandparent) had either supplemented formal care, or been used before formal care began. In fact, some family members used strong statements to describe formal childcare, reflecting distrust and even hostility (e.g. 'dumped in nurseries'; 'sling it [child] out to a childminder'). There was frequent use of terms such as 'strangers' and 'outsiders' when referring to formal carers.

Similar views about informal care being preferable to formal care were also expressed in relation to older people. Carers interviewed in the Fifty Plus study spoke about the reluctance of their parents to accept formal services and support from outside the family. As with childcare, terms such as 'outsiders' and 'strangers' were used to describe formal carers. Perhaps the resistance to formal services is due to an understandable reluctance among older people to acknowledge that they can no longer manage independently. This is a particularly sensitive issue when older generations, who see themselves as the senior members of the family and who have traditionally given support to younger generations, find themselves in a position of dependency (Finch 1989).

However, there is some evidence that views and preferences are starting to change, with the next generation of older people more likely to demand and expect formal care services (Brookes et al. 2002). In the Four Generation study, the expressed preference for informal care was less strong among younger generations than their parents and grandparents. Even among the older generations (grandparents and great grandparents), some did not expect to be cared for by their children and grandchildren in the way that they themselves had cared for older generations. There was a tendency to talk more about independence and not becoming a burden to their children. As this grandfather put it,

> [I] wouldn't expect to go and live with one of them. I would want them all to keep in touch, and to lend their support and to visit, but I don't think it would be fair to expect any more than that. So, if I couldn't do [care] for myself, and [wife] wasn't here, I guess I'd be looking for some

kind of professional help. Um, maybe in my own home, maybe in a – in a home where I'm cared for.

The desire not to see their own children caring for them in the same way that they themselves were caring for their parents was also spontaneously commented upon by many of the informal carers in the Fifty Plus study. This was perhaps because they were currently experiencing the impact of taking on the responsibility of caring for someone, or had recently done so.

> There's no way that I would ever say that I did what I did because it was duty, I did it because he was my dad, he was my friend, and that's fine – but I would not ever choose for my children to be in that position . . . it's not just that I've got heartless uncaring children . . . but if I really felt I was going to be dependent on my children in the same way I would jump off a bridge or something because it is stressful, it is a strain.

Availability and adequacy of formal care services

Formal services can relieve relatives of some of the pressure of caring and undertaking personal care, as recognised by English elder care workers when talking about the benefits of such services (Johansson and Moss 2004). Providing intimate care for a close relative such as a parent can be particularly difficult. Both men and women in the Fifty Plus study talked about what was appropriate care for them to provide. For example, although the husband of one interviewee provided much support for his mother, it was his wife not he who helped with his mother's personal care needs such as bathing. Formal services can offer high quality care and close relationships, but without the same emotional intensity of family relationships. It was apparent in some accounts in the Fifty Plus study that the relationship between carer and care recipient could induce feelings of guilt, about not doing enough or neglecting other close family members, and, implicit if not explicit, at times a feeling of being manipulated by the person receiving care. This led one female carer to conclude that formal care might be preferable because 'there's not the emotional ties and the sort of emotional strings that can be pulled'.

But formal care services were not always available, or acceptable to families. Some carers interviewed in the two studies felt that they had little choice over becoming an informal carer, because there was simply no-one else to do it either within or outside the family. Many carers in the Fifty Plus study, for example, spoke about the inadequacies of formal services for supporting elderly parents: 'I'm actually appalled, I really didn't realize that there was so little available, and the hoops that you have to jump through to get it.' Formal services were sometimes rejected because of a perception of poor quality, or because they would not be accepted by the person needing care. Interviewees in the Four Generation study, such as the grandmother and grandfather quoted below, talked about their experiences of the availability and quality of formal services and its influence on their decision-making:

> It's dreadful care, the Social Services . . . My poor old Auntie Flo, she died round on that geriatric ward at [hospital] . . . I don't care if I have to give up my job, everything. I wouldn't put my mum anywhere like that. Ain't leaving *her* to the tender mercies of the Social Services.

> I've had to look after mine, they'll have to look after me . . . I mean, I wouldn't want to be chucked in an old people's home. I've seen enough old people's homes when I worked on the Council. I'd rather be dead than stuck in one of them places.

In the case of childcare, a decision to use informal care could also reflect the lack of accessible and affordable formal care rather than a real preference for this type of provision.

Surveys have shown that 85 per cent of working mothers would like to use some formal childcare (i.e. childminders, nurseries, preschool playgroups and out-of-school clubs) if it were readily available and affordable (Woodland et al. 2002). Although there has been a substantial increase in government spending and expansion of the childcare sector, more than a quarter of all families still report not being able to find a formal childcare place when they need it (Woodland et al. 2002). There are also important differences between families in their use of formal and informal childcare. Use of formal services is higher among parents who work full time, who are in higher earning jobs and who are living as a couple (Mooney et al. 2001). Lone parents, parents working part time and parents in lower earning jobs are more likely to use informal childcare. So are parents who work at atypical times such as weekends, overnight or shift work. Formal childcare services rarely cover such times, and these parents usually need to rely on informal carers such as partners, ex-partners and grandparents to meet their childcare needs (La Valle et al. 2002; Statham and Mooney 2003).

The impact of providing informal care

Having considered the reasons why people do (or do not) provide informal care, we turn finally to the impact that providing such care can have on the carer. It is important to begin by drawing a distinction between informal childcare and informal care for the elderly, sick or disabled. Childcare is time limited and the hours are usually predictable. Primary responsibility for the child's welfare remains with their parents. Other forms of informal care are less predictable and its course and duration less certain. For example, care may be intermittent, such as helping a relative over a crisis with little involvement until the next crisis episode; or it can gradually grow until the carer is fully responsible for the person's welfare. Alternatively, care can begin suddenly with little warning, for example with the diagnosis of a chronic illness or the death of one parent leaving the surviving parent needing more help or support.

Four categories of carer have been distinguished: 'major carers' who provide regular care that is considerably demanding of their time; 'semi-carers' who help with such tasks as shopping and cleaning; 'monitoring carers' who may need to visit regularly and 'keep an eye on things'; and short-term 'crisis carers', usually associated with recovery after hospitalisation or serious illness (Watson and Mears 1999). These different levels of care require different levels of emotional and physical involvement and affect carers in different ways.

One further point needs to be made, which concerns the difference in looking after young children and in looking after older people. Whereas both childcare and eldercare can be rewarding, eldercare may at times be less so, particularly when one is witnessing the increasing frailty and dependency of a loved one. Unlike eldercare, there was little negative feeling expressed about childcare for grandchildren in the Fifty Plus study. Those who were combining care of a grandchild and an elderly parent could find this particularly stressful.

Here a retired grandmother from this study expresses her feelings about caring for her grandchildren and her father: 'I love having the grandchildren. I don't find it onerous at all. I love my dad and I want to support him, but I can't say it's always a pleasure. There's lots of times when it is a pleasure, but lots of times when it's difficult.'

The effects of providing informal care can be negative or positive, and sometimes both. One in seven of the carers surveyed in the Fifty Plus study reported that providing care was both satisfying and stressful. On the one hand, there is the reassurance that the person is well looked after and the satisfaction of helping and giving something back to loved ones. On the other hand, there are the stresses and strains of coping with illness, physical frailty or disability, particularly if there is inadequate support from formal services, as seemed to be the case for many of the carers we interviewed. There is also the added difficulty of coming to terms with a reversal of roles when parents become more dependent on their adult children. Caring responsibilities can make life more stressful and leave less time for families and for the carers themselves, and these effects are felt more as the number of care hours increases (Table 9.2). When carers are combining informal care with paid work, the pressure and resulting stress can affect relationships at home. As a carer in the Fifty Plus study explained, 'there wasn't enough of me to go round', and this sometimes led to impatience, less time for partners, and feeling less relaxed at home.

Working lives could also be affected, through needing to find time to make phone calls to formal agencies and services, having to take longer lunch breaks to make hospital visits or dash back home to check on someone, or being unable to increase working hours. Concentration could also be

Table 9.2 How hours of care affect carers

	<5 hours (n = 173) %	5–19 hours (n = 172) %	20+ hours (n = 104) %	Total (n = 449) %
Makes life more stressful	31	54	60	47
Less time for self	15	49	58	39
Less time for family	16	42	46	33

Source: Fifty Plus study

Note: Multiple response question therefore columns total more than 100%.

affected. A learning support assistant working part time described how her care responsibilities affected her concentration span: 'I was sitting thinking about my mum and dad and my daughter and . . . I mean when you're working with Special Needs children you've got to be focused.' Such difficulties did not necessarily mean that employees were unable to do their job properly. Rather, it placed them under additional stress that affected them in other ways, particularly their health and their ability to progress in their careers. For example, a senior planning officer and father interviewed in the Fifty Plus study, whose daughter had a severe learning disability, had not pursued promotion because of the additional stress a new job would bring: 'If you've got a stressful job at work and then go home and it's stressful it takes its toll . . . I mean, I feel I can cope with the stresses here and the stresses at home because I know the ropes here.'

A mother with secondary school-aged children who worked as a part-time school secretary was unable to further her career, in part because of caring for her elderly mother: 'I love what I do and am excited by new ideas, but feel unable to put myself forward for further training because I cannot give the best of myself.' Her head teacher had asked if she would like to increase her hours, but 'I knew I just could not do it along with everything else. I would love to give more of myself to the school. I know it's thought I don't give enough free time to concerts and events, but I just have not got the time.'

Forgoing career advancement and being unable to increase part-time hours have significant financial implications. One mother with two adult sons, working full time in a senior post in the local authority youth service and with care responsibilities for her mother, explained why she would be unlikely to seek promotion:

And you know at 53 would I want to be taking on all of that when, you know, my mum being in her very late 70s – you've got to be realistic about this and thinking that something is likely to happen in the not too distant future and how would that affect it? Whereas the other side of it is, pension-wise, if I was to take on another senior role then the pension would go up. So in the end on balance I decided no, I wouldn't apply for it and didn't . . . But I can see that if I didn't have the responsibility of my mother then you know . . . then there would have been nothing to stop me going for it.

Conclusions: the future of informal care

Informal care, as with formal care, involves meeting a diverse range of physical, emotional and practical needs, whether for children or older adults. Both formal and informal care is highly gendered. With eldercare, women are more likely to be the primary caregiver, to do more hours of care and to be more involved in intimate care compared with men. With childcare, grandmothers tend to be the main carer though grandfathers may support them. The distinguishing features of informal care are that it is usually unpaid, unregulated and largely based on family obligations and reciprocity, which are often transmitted across generations.

There is significant use of care provided by family, friends and neighbours, though it is difficult to know how, in the light of improved services, the use of informal care would change. A preference for informal care and a distrust of 'stranger' care both for children and older adults is apparent, although this appears to be changing among younger generations and again has to be seen within the context of a lack of formal provision that would allow a true choice. On the supply side, there perhaps is growing reluctance among grandparents to provide full-time childcare for their grandchildren, and recognition among parent and grandparent generations that grandparents should be allowed to enjoy their leisure time. Although caregiving can be rewarding it can also have negative consequences, particularly eldercare. These negative effects include stress, ill health, less time for the carer and their immediate family. For those in paid work, it can reduce employment opportunities.

What is the future likely to hold for informal care? Given the apparent preference for this form of care and the importance of reciprocity and family obligations identified in our studies, one could argue it is likely to remain significant. However, there are a number of social and demographic changes underway that may influence both the demand for, and supply of, informal care.

Significant changes in recent decades in birth and morbidity rates, in the age of first childbirth and in maternal employment are influencing the demand for childcare and eldercare. Demographically, families are smaller and people are living longer. In the Four Generation study, for example, the parent generation (with a child under age 10 in 1999) came from much smaller families than the great-grandparent generation, and were the only generation in which some participants grew up as only children. This has led to what has become known as beanpole families: more surviving generations, but with fewer members in each one. Sixty-two per cent of grandparents in the British Social Attitudes Survey were not the senior generation in their family, which could have four, five or even six generations (Dench and Ogg 2002). Other surveys report that one third of those aged 80 or over are members of four-generation families, as are one fifth of those aged 20 to 29 and 50 to 59 and a quarter of those in their thirties (Grundy et al. 1999).

With increased longevity, it is estimated that people aged 75 or over will increase by over 70 per cent in the next 30 years or so (Carers UK 2001). The number of people aged between 45 and 65 – those most likely to provide care – is estimated to rise by only 11 per cent over the same period. Thus, although the potential requirement for help with daily living is set to increase, the number of people who might provide such help is forecast to decrease. Women in their fifties and sixties, who have traditionally been the main providers of kin care (Hutton and Hirst 1999; McKay and Middleton 1998), are increasingly being attracted into, or remaining in, the paid workforce. During the 1980s and 1990s, the proportion of women in this age group who were working rose, whilst the proportion of working men in the same age group decreased (Mooney et al. 2002). Working hours have also risen, particularly for women in their early fifties. There is evidence to suggest that increasing employment among women may account for the decline in intensive caregiving (50 hours or more a week) for older parents and parents-in-law (Pickard 2002).

Another factor contributing to increased demand for care services is the significant increase in the employment of women with a young child, from just over a quarter of women with a child under age 5 being in paid work in 1980 to more than half in 2002 (Office for National Statistics 2003c). The dominant family model of one parent working full time and the other staying at home is no longer the norm, if indeed it ever was. Children are now more likely to live in households where both parents work, though usually one full time and one part time.

Taken together, these demographic and labour market changes have a number of possible consequences. First, grandparents will be older and may be less able to provide childcare for young grandchildren. Second, there is an increasing likelihood that these grandparents will be caught between the competing demands for care from both younger and older generations, particularly as a result of increased longevity. Finally, the responsibility for elderly people will increasingly fall on kin who are of working age. Older women are more likely now to be working, and to be working longer hours. Our findings suggest that this generation of women often do not want to give up work to become full-time carers. Future generations of grandmothers with higher levels of education, better jobs and fewer if any employment breaks may be even less willing to leave employment in their fifties to take on care responsibilities. They may also be unable to afford to do so. The growing pension crisis means that both men and women are likely to have to continue working to an older age in order to fund their retirement, and will thus be less available to provide care (Evandrou 2003).

Other factors may conspire to weaken family relationships and family obligations. We know that geographic proximity is important in determining the extent that family members are able to provide direct help to one another. Families may become more dispersed due to job relocation and the search for affordable housing by the younger generation. Increased geographical mobility together with the time-bind that many families find themselves in may make it difficult to maintain relationships with the wider family, although research suggests that the conditions in which contemporary families find themselves have altered but not weakened the commitments that people make (Williams 2004).

Demand for informal care may also be affected by an expansion in the provision of formal care. Would more childcare services, for example, eliminate the need or desire for informal childcare? There is evidence from other countries to suggest that formal services do not displace informal care, but rather that the nature of informal care changes as formal care services become widely available (Van Ewijk et al. 2002b). In Sweden, where affordable childcare is widely available, there is very little use of informal care on a regular basis, but grandparents play a role in helping out in an emergency. With respect to eldercare, informal carers such as relatives may re-shape their role into one of organising and brokering formal services, acting as an advocate for the person being cared for, and providing emotional support rather than undertaking the routine practical tasks of caring.

Finally, it is important that informal care is not viewed in isolation from the availability and acceptability of formal care services: both are required. In line with the conclusions of a study of social care in five European countries, including England (Sipila and Kroger 2004), we would argue that affordable formal care services need to be seen as the backbone of social care, enabling families to have real choice in their lives.

> If the whole care arrangement is based only on an informal caregiving network, human relationships come under constant strain and may break down unexpectedly. The time and space created by social care services allow women in particular to make individual choices about how they live and work. Last but not least, formal services regulate the working conditions of caregivers whereas informal care can often in practice mean exploitation of a person who is in a weak social position.
>
> (Sipilä and Kröger 2004: 562)

Our own and others' research has shown that many people have a strong commitment and desire to care for others, and this moral 'ethic of care' needs to be developed and fostered as a counter-balance to the current emphasis on an 'ethic of work' (Watson and Mears 1999; Williams 2001).

Strategies are needed to increase the availability of formal care services, both as an alternative to and as a support for informal care; to develop family-friendly employment practices; and to encourage a more equal sharing of caring responsibilities between men and women. Such a view was well expressed by one of the participants in the Fifty Plus study:

> I think that we need to look at the whole situation of the family in the broader context and just recognise that everybody has needs and those needs should be met. And it shouldn't be down to individuals to go and beg for half hours off, hours off . . . we should have a far more inclusive situation so that these should just be somebody's right. If I have a need to take a grandchild somewhere, to take a parent somewhere, to take a husband somewhere, then I think that should be my right.

Notes

1 All names have been anonymised.
2 Each of the three generations interviewed for the Four Generation study are referred to by their relationship to the fourth and youngest generation: parent, grandparent and great-grandparent.

10 The future of care work

*Peter Moss, Claire Cameron, and
Janet Boddy*

In the preceding chapters we have looked at various facets of the present
state of care work, across historical time and the life course and from
informal care by relatives to the highly professionalised work of the
pedagogue with a variety of points in between. In this concluding chapter we
look to the future, picking up on some of the issues we raised in our introduction and which have emerged in subsequent chapters. We start by offering
some answers to two key questions. Does care work have a future? Is there a
crisis in care work? We conclude by considering what form or shape care
work – paid or unpaid – might take over the first part of this century.

Our answers are, of course, highly provisional. We have seen the fluidity
and variability of care work from a historical and cultural perspective, and
discussed how the work is shaped and understood within particular historical
and cultural contexts. As these contexts change, so too do structures and
understandings. Nor can we begin to tell what the context for care work will
be in 30, let alone 50 or 100 years, any more than writers in 1900 could have
imagined the world in 1950 or 1999. We suspect, and very much hope, that
care of our environment will have become an absolute global priority,
reminding us of Tronto's inclusive definition of care as 'a species activity
that includes everything that we do to maintain, continue and repair our
"world" so we can live in it as well as possible. That world includes our
bodies, our selves, and our environment, all of which we seek to interweave
in a complex, life sustaining web' (1993: 8).

However, because we cannot know and be certain does not mean that we
should not be thinking about the future, especially when it comes to an issue
of such great importance to all of us as individuals and to the societies of
which we are members. From this perspective we find it strange how little
strategic attention is paid by the UK government to imagining the big future
picture of care, at a time when so many of the assumptions and foundations
on which care work has been based are questioned and crumbling. This
neglect is thrown into sharp relief when contrasted with the work of the UK
Ministry of Defence in conducting an ongoing review of Strategic Trends,
described as 'an ambitious attempt to develop a coherent view of how the
world might develop over the next thirty years in ways that could alter

the UK's security . . . [the analysis being] broken down into seven Dimensions, the Physical, Social [including family life], Science and Technology, Economic, Legal, Political and Military' (Ministry of Defence 2005).[1]

So if we venture one recommendation it would be that government, in partnership with a wide range of civil society organisations, undertakes a similar rolling exercise with respect to the future prospects for care – not just one department looking at one area of policy interest (be it childcare, residential care, foster care, social care), but a cross-departmental and cross-societal exercise linking care in all its forms with demography, employment, gender and community.

Does care work have a future?

The answer to this question is yes and no. Yes, in the sense that there will be a continuing need for the varied and extensive activities that we talk about today in policy and everyday language as 'care'. 'Care' is the bedrock of any society, without which it can neither function nor be a fit place to live. But no, in the narrower sense that we question whether 'care' should continue to be treated as a separate field for policy and employment purposes.

Our doubts on this score arise for the two reasons we set out in chapter 1. First, because 'care' is often weakly conceptualised in policy – there is little clarity about what 'care' means, leaving it badly positioned to defend its separate identity. As we argued in chapter 1, terms like 'social care' or 'childcare' are, in practice, little more than labels for groups of services and workers arbitrarily linked together in a single policy field, at a particular moment of time. Second, and related, in the search for services that are more 'joined up' and for workers who can address the whole person, the borders between 'care' and other policy and employment areas are blurring and crumbling – for example, between childcare and education, or between adult social care, health and housing. Taking this a step further, as discussed in chapter 6, there is already a well-established 'generic' theory and practice found in much of continental Europe which subsumes care into a holistic approach to working with people – pedagogy. Of course the same rationale could be applied to other areas of policy and employment, requiring either new, more encompassing concepts or the redefinition of existing concepts – 'education' for example to be understood as 'education in its broadest sense'.

But the passing of 'care' as a concept that defines and structures policy and employment would not mean the end of care in policy and employment; no longer to have a distinct policy and employment field labelled 'care' does not mean being care-less in practice. Indeed, arguably, 'care' should feature more widely and explicitly, as a value throughout all areas of policy and employment. Herein lies the potential power of the concept of the 'ethics of care', with its mixture of 'particular acts of caring and a "general habit of mind" to care that should inform all aspects of moral life' (Tronto

1993: 127), care combining a disposition (made up of responsibility, competence, integrity and responsiveness) and certain actions. Working with this concept – of care as an ethic – we could ask whether or not a nursery, a school, a hospital, a university, a nursing home, a prison, a benefit office, a telephone helpline, or any other environment where policy is implemented, works with this ethic, and whether or not the staff in these organisations display care. In this sense, we can all be viewed as potential 'care workers', but with no one having a job description confined to care.

(Although we are doubtful about the future of 'care work' as a term defining a distinct policy and employment field, we continue to use the term in the remainder of this chapter, to cover the broad field that has been the subject of this book, including unpaid work. This is partly to avoid confusion and partly because alternative terms are lacking or – as in the case of 'pedagogical work' – unfamiliar to readers in the English-language world.)

Is care work in crisis?

Again, the answer is both yes and no. Yes, in the sense that the present state of affairs looks likely to be unsustainable. As we discussed in the introduction, demand for care work is increasing at the very moment when the usual sources of supply – paid and unpaid – are decreasing, and we repeat the warning offered by Coomans (2002):

> wherever the present standard for any category of job is 'low qualified women around the age of 30', there will unmistakably be a strong need to improve the quality of job so it will be acceptable to people with higher educational attainments. And if no improved professionalisation of the job was achieved, then it will rapidly end up in a severe labour supply shortage.

The situation in Britain is acute because, as we have seen in several chapters, many care workers have low levels of qualification and are paid badly, while low skilled jobs in other less demanding sectors are available. The promised labour shortages are already appearing, with increasing problems of recruitment and retention of paid workers: 'social care has been one of the fastest growing sectors of the economy in modern times ... As such, social care providers face ongoing challenges of recruitment and retention, heightened due to competition between statutory, private and voluntary care workers, as well as education and the National Health Service ... The evidence suggests demand and expectations will continue to grow, and as such will put greater demands on the social care labour market' (Roche and Rankin 2004: 6). Similar comments could be made about childcare and other care work sectors.

But the present state of affairs will not continue, for as we have seen the history of care work is one of fluidity, change and evolution. In our view, therefore, systems of service provision will adjust to avert full crisis. But in what ways? And who will end up doing care work? Under what conditions? And who will pay?

There are various possible answers to these questions and the process of deciding from among them is highly political. There are also more practical issues involved, not least the actual viability of proposed solutions. Here we will sketch out a few possibilities, though in practice some sort of hybrid solution – mixing some, all or other solutions – is likely to emerge.

Keeping care in the family   Policies can support existing informal patterns of care by family members – for children and adults with disabilities. Maternity and parental leave entitlements are one example of such policies, as are cash for care or direct payment schemes which allow relatives to be 'employed' by people needing care. Viability here concerns whether it is possible to reverse trends, especially in employment (for example, more women working, later retirement of women and men), that affect patterns of informal care. Can informal care be strengthened and, if so, under what conditions and with what consequences on other societal objectives?

The 'third sector' workforce   Since 1997, the current UK government has emphasised the role of the voluntary sector in public service provision, as part of policies towards 'active citizenship'. Chapter 7 provides one example of how government has sought to pursue this goal and the distinctive role that volunteers can play. The viability issue here is similar to keeping care in the family – how do you create space for voluntary care work in a world which increasingly requires 'active citizens' to be employed and earning?

Searching for new labour reserves   Policies can be introduced to boost recruitment from under-represented groups in the workforce, for example men, particular age groups, or people with disabilities. This may be part of a general approach to develop a more diverse national labour force in all occupations and at all levels of qualification; or it may be a more focused search for new supplies of low qualified applicants, for example through 'welfare to work' policies which identify care work as a priority area for the employment of previously unemployed or economically inactive women and men with few if any academic or vocational qualifications. One viability issue concerns timescale: men represent the largest potential but untapped labour reserve for the care workforce, but change here, while possible, is likely to be a long-term project. Another issue concerns the level of education and qualification expected of the future care worker, an issue we discuss below. 'Welfare to work' arguments can readily assume continuing low entry requirements for care work: but this assumption is not consistent with an increasing recognition that a well-educated workforce is needed to ensure high standards of work.

Migrant labour   Many public services in London (social work, nursing, teaching) already depend to a greater or lesser extent on migrant labour. The same is true, more globally, for certain forms of private domestic work with a large care component (within a week of each other, in late 2004, both the UK Home Secretary and the US President's candidate for the post of Secretary for Homeland Security resigned over questions about possible misdemeanours involving the employment of migrant workers as nannies). The future might involve increasing use of migrant labour, both well-qualified workers (for example, nursery and kindergarten workers from Central and Eastern Europe for 'childcare' services in the UK) and less qualified workers (for example, for domiciliary and residential care services for older people). Viability here is bound up with wider issues concerning national policy on migrant labour and recognition of overseas qualifications. But there is also a more specific issue of the need for migrant care workers to have a working knowledge of English which may be a problem for many with lower levels of education.

Revaluing and reconceptualising the work   'Care work', in part or overall, can be revalued, in terms of qualification, pay and employment conditions, to make it more attractive and better able to hold its own in the labour market. This strategy has been followed in a number of countries with respect, for example, to early childhood services. In these services, the Nordic countries have moved to a graduate worker accounting for at least half the workforce (either a pedagogue or, in the recent case of Sweden, a teacher); while New Zealand, as part of a reform process which has defined these services as 'early childhood education' (education in this case viewed in its broadest sense), is committed to all staff in most types of early childhood services having an early years teaching qualification by 2012 backed up by pay parity across the whole teaching workforce (i.e. teachers will earn the same whether working with 18-month-olds or 18-year-olds). As these examples indicate, when 'care work' is revalued it usually stops being conceptualised and termed 'care work': in the countries just referred to, what is 'childcare' in the UK is part of 'pedagogy' or 'education'. A question remains, therefore, whether work explicitly described and understood as 'just' care can escape the low social valuation and recognition that attaches to such work at present. Viability in this case centrally involves issues of cost, since revaluing involves a substantial increase in funding for the work: as far as we know, there are no examples of widespread revaluing of care work being financed by users, through market mechanisms, so this possibility requires more public expenditure.

Underlying the putative crisis of care, and running as a connecting thread through the chapters of this book, is gender. The crisis facing care work arises from the fact that the work – whether undertaken by paid workers, unpaid relatives or volunteers such as mentors – is heavily gendered, being disproportionately undertaken by women: we have seen this in almost every chapter of the book. The gendered nature of unpaid work in the family has spilled over into paid work, where the imbalance has been reproduced; indeed, today paid care work is more gendered than unpaid care work.

In our view, the main reasons for the gendering of paid care work are not, as often assumed, low pay and bad employment conditions. These are effects rather than causes. Consequently, the workforce remains highly gendered even in cases where 'care work' has been revalued as in early childhood services in the Nordic countries; while individual cases of 'gender mixed' training and employment in early childhood work have been achieved despite low levels of pay.

The heart of the matter, in our view, lies in how care work has, over time, become understood as work for which women are essentially best suited, by dint of innate qualities or acquired domestic skills: care work is, in short, seen as women's work and is low paid because it is associated with an activity that women 'naturally' know how to do. The gendering of the work-force is then reproduced and reinforced through training and employment regimes that assume, and are structured to provide for, a corps of female students and workers.

The problem facing all post-industrial societies is that care work can no longer depend on women assuming the greater part of the associated work and costs. Gender roles, relationships and expectations have changed radic-ally and rapidly, so that 'in the last generations, it has become more difficult to maintain the fictional separations of public and private life because it has become more clear, especially as women have been more fully included in public life, how this separation is artificial' (Tronto 2004: 1). A system of care that assumed women would leave employment to provide care or that they could be relied on to provide low paid care work, often part time, because it was compatible with their own care responsibilities is breaking down as women's educational levels equal and surpass those of men, as women's employment careers come to look more like men's, and as partici-pation in the labour market will have to extend longer, well into the sixties, to ensure an adequate retirement pension.

So far, however, most economic and social institutions (including govern-ment, workplaces and public services) have failed to acknowledge and confront the scale of these changes and their implications. There is increas-ing talk about 'work/life' balance, but this scratches the surface rather than disturbing what lies beneath. This is very clear in the UK. Attempts are made to give women more 'flexibility' in their employment, without questioning the basic structures of employment and the assumptions underpinning them (i.e. making continuous full-time employment the normative pattern of work, which is necessary for career progression and a financially secure retirement); fathers are given two weeks' low-paid paternity leave, but the extent and nature of the changes required of men in providing care of children or others is little discussed and, at the same time, the introduction of a year's maternity leave sends a message that women are primarily responsible for the care of very young children; modest targets are set for male workers in childcare services, but the strategic and cross-sectoral issue of who will work with children and old people in the future remains unaddressed.

Like all crises, the impending crisis of care is not necessarily a catastrophe or even a problem. By forcing us to think and question, rather than continuing to take things for granted, it can open up to new possibilities: the possibility, for example, of men and women engaging equally in home and workplace, care becoming men's as well as women's work; and the possibility of a better society which gives equal value to care relations and entrepreneurial activity. But first the crisis needs to be acknowledged, and the reasons for it appreciated.

Some future possibilities for care work

We will end with some reflections on possible future directions for care work itself, less as an exercise in prediction than as a contribution to the wide-ranging discussion that we have argued is necessitated by the impending crisis of care. We consider both paid and unpaid care work, not only to recognise that work is not confined to employment, but because the two fields are connected in many ways – changes in one will affect the other, just as participation in one type of work may affect participation in the other. Our reflections are informed by the range of studies undertaken at the Thomas Coram Research Unit in recent years and especially by the recently completed study 'Care Work in Europe', which has been both cross-national and cross-sectoral, covering work with children, young people and adults both younger and older.

Two conclusions from that study form a starting point for these reflections. Both raise questions about the rationale for and necessity of the segmentation of *paid* care work in many countries, that is the dividing off of the workforce into different occupations with different qualifications working with different groups often defined in terms of age. The first conclusion is that care work in all sectors is complex and demanding work and requires certain *shared* abilities and competences including the ability to:

- reflect and make contextualised judgements;
- communicate, listen and network;
- support inclusion and citizenship;
- work with complexity, diversity, change;
- adopt a holistic approach;
- support development, learning and autonomy;
- combine theory and practice.

Second, the study concluded that care workers, again in all sectors, are facing new understandings or images of the people with whom they are working. Whether very young children or very old adults, there is a turn to viewing 'users' no longer as passive objects and dependents but as active subjects and citizens with rights. This makes the work both more demanding and more interesting.

Such conclusions support the case for better educated workers (already widely accepted in the UK policy discourse) but also for considering more generic occupations, cutting across sectors and groups. They also question why, as at present, care workers with children are better educated than those with older people and why care workers in general have lower levels of education than, say, teachers, nurses or social workers. Such reflections are further provoked by the experience of Denmark (discussed for example in chapter 6), where 'care work' across a wide range of the life course is based on a generic and graduate level worker, the pedagogue (with some discussion about extending the work of the pedagogue into elder care, pedagogues themselves claiming they are equipped to work with people from birth to 100!).

So one direction in the UK might be to develop a new generic profession in care work, which might be the pedagogue but could be some other 'made in the UK' hybrid profession (although, if the pedagogue was adopted as this profession, this would mean rethinking 'care work' as 'pedagogical work', with the added advantage that this is a concept with a long tradition and a well-developed theory and practice). What we are envisaging here is a profession which can span the current policy divide between, on the one hand, work with children and young people (now in England and Scotland located in education departments) and adult 'social care' (located in health and welfare). We are, therefore, proposing to go *beyond* current discussions, for example in England, that seek a common core of skills, knowledge and competence for the 'widest possible range of workers in children's services' (Department for Education and Skills 2003), both because we propose going beyond shared elements of training across existing occupations to a new profession that subsumes many occupations, and because that profession would go beyond work in children's services to work across services for children and adults.

This would in turn generate other questions. For example, what relationship would this new profession have with other existing professions, such as teachers, social workers, therapists and nurses? Who, for example, would work in early childhood services – the new profession, teachers or both? What areas of work would be included within the boundaries of this new profession and where would the boundary be pitched?

Another question would be what place this new profession would occupy in the entire workforce of the services in which the profession worked, and who would make up the remainder of that workforce? One view would envisage the new generic professional making up a thin but broad layer spanning many services, providing a managerial, supervisory and/or senior practitioner position, while leaving the direct, front-line work to a less educated group of workers (see Van Ewijk 2005). Thus, for example, this new generic professional might be the head of a service for older people or a residential service for young people, whilst the everyday work with the older or young people would be left to workers with a lower level of qualification. Another view, more akin to the Danish use of pedagogues, would see the new professional making up a large part of the workforce, including many of those doing direct front-line work where they would work alongside (and not simply above) a group of less educated workers.

The former approach would be argued on grounds of cost, but also on grounds of the nature of the work. Direct work with people, the rationale would go, involves performing a range of discrete tasks, following laid-down procedures and achieving predefined outcomes. This does not require a graduate and professional practitioner, but rather a hierarchy of vocationally trained technicians, capable of operating to industry-defined standards in the performance of their range of tasks.

The latter approach necessitates a different understanding of the work. The professional-as-frontline-worker would be argued on grounds of the complex nature of the work and the abilities needed to do it, as well as a pedagogical view of the work as essentially relational and holistic. Put at its most basic, from this perspective blowing someone's nose or washing someone are not simply discrete tasks that can be delegated to a person with training in nose blowing and washing; they are necessary parts of relating to the other person, who cannot be viewed as a collection of separable parts and needs. When I blow someone's nose or wash them I do so as part of a relationship and these actions develop and deepen that relationship and create opportunities for supporting that person's development, inclusion and autonomy. Moreover, this higher educated worker, while capable of following procedures and striving towards predefined outcomes, would have the ability to apply contextualised judgements. She or he would be able to work with, even thrive on, uncertainty and provisionality and could see how practice needs to take account of context, typified perhaps in the phrase 'it depends . . .' (for a discussion of uncertainty as a value, see Rinaldi 2005). Through reflection on specific situations and dialogue with service users and others, the professional front-line worker would be open to recognising and appreciating outcomes that were not previously anticipated but which might be of great value.

Whatever the type and extent of the more highly educated worker, there seems little argument that all paid workers need education, and should have the opportunity, if they wish, to undertake further education to qualify as a pedagogue (or however the higher educated worker is defined). Our assumption therefore is that the future of paid care involves an expanding and better educated workforce. What we are less certain about is how this broad trend may relate to, or be affected by, another trend: the growing use of direct payments by adult care users to employ people to provide them with the support they need for independent living. This trend brings together two elements that, potentially, could weaken the position of the paid care worker: working in a domestic setting which, as we saw in chapter 5, raises particular ambiguities and tensions; and the 'personal assistant' being accountable wholly to the care user who, for example, in some schemes at least, may assess their assistants' training needs. With the expansion of direct payment schemes very much on the table in many countries, the implications of an increasingly well-educated workforce and increasing user power require urgent consideration.

What implications does an expanding paid care workforce have for unpaid care work, either involving family members or friends or people volunteering their time, as for example mentors or foster parents? We should return first of all to a rather more complex concept than a simple paid/unpaid dichotomy, to the idea which we raised in chapter 1 of a care work continuum defined in terms of status and formality, ranging from informal family carers to the profession of pedagogue. As we suggested then, types of care work are spread along this continuum and change positions on it as different aspects of each type of work change – as, for example, not only payment but regulation, education and status vary. Unpaid work like mentoring may move along the continuum as it becomes more regulated, develops qualifications and systems of accreditation and perhaps moves to a position where some mentors are paid while others still serve as volunteers; the position of foster care could similarly alter. Thus, change does not simply involve going from one state (unpaid work) to another (paid work); it is a more complex process, involving changes in an assemblage of dimensions that move the work to a greater or lesser extent along the continuum.

Another problem with a simple paid/unpaid dichotomy is that it reproduces misleading notions that work which moves from the home to a public setting remains essentially the same, the only differences being who does the work, where it is done (in some cases) and who pays. Instead, we would argue that when work moves from, say, the family to being conducted, say, in an institution or by a paid worker, there are important changes too in its relationships, practices and, sometimes, purposes. Pedagogues, teachers, childcare workers in nurseries and family day carers are not substitute mothers, nor are the settings in which they work substitute homes: they are qualitatively different experiences. These experiences bring both risks and possibilities.

We do not see that a broad movement towards a better educated and paid workforce means the tapering off or end of other forms of care work, whether by family and friends or by volunteers. It would neither be feasible nor in the least desirable for all care work to be paid work; unpaid care work has an important role to play both today and in the future. However, attention does need to be paid to the conditions needed for unpaid care work to flourish, rather than for it to be a source of stress and disadvantage to those who undertake it.

This issue – how unpaid care work may flourish – becomes more acute in a society where increasing value is placed on paid employment and which expects 'autonomous citizens' to assume increasing responsibility for managing their own and family members' risks. Costs – for example, pensions and higher education – are increasingly privatised, to be paid for from individual's employment earnings. In this process, the person who leaves or reduces employment either to care for family or friends or to take up voluntary care work finds themselves at an increasing disadvantage, both at the time and subsequently, right through into retirement. The same applies to women or men who wish to give more time to other forms of voluntary work in civil society, for example, participating in local democratic politics or becoming a school or hospital governor.

We think the forward look on care work that we recommended at the start of this chapter needs to envisage bold and imaginative possibilities. For paid work, this might involve the development of good quality employment across the care work field, including perhaps an extensive generic profession crossing current borders and sectors. For unpaid work, it might involve major rethinking about working life, going well beyond leave policies focused on narrow phases of the life course (notably maternity and parental leave limited to early parenthood) to wide-ranging 'time account' schemes giving women and men quotas of time they can take away from employment – across the life course, for many reasons, and on either full-time or part-time bases. This should be linked to rethinking pensions, so that women and men have access to funding for when they are not working, be it while taking career breaks or during retirement (which will almost certainly start at later ages as the century proceeds). It should also be linked to active measures to encourage men as well as women to take breaks for care reasons, for without this the 'male employment career' model will continue to be normative and policies to give workers more non-employment time will become yet more pitfalls on the road to gender equality.

But we might need to go even further, to link time account schemes to a new concept of what Beck calls 'public work', a 'new focus of activity and identity that will revitalize the democratic way of life' (1998: 60). The concept covers activities that Beck divides under three headings: active compassion (including what we have termed volunteer care work); practical critique (in which people use their professional skills in different settings); and active democracy (citizen participation in decentralised politics and services). What this means, Beck argues, is that we have to invest in civil society:

> In the future what will probably win out is a blending of formal work and voluntary organisation, the dismantling of legal and mobility barriers between the two sectors, the creation of opportunities for leaving or changing one's principal occupation (in an annual, monthly or weekly rhythm) ... The material and cultural foundations for 'individualism coupled with solidarity' would be established.
>
> (ibid.)

He concludes his discussion of 'public works' by exploring who would pay for a system which valued voluntary work, suggesting three possibilities: tax reductions for those engaging in public work; a tax-based basic support payment for those doing public work; or citizens' support for all, a sort of universal minimum income.

The question of who pays haunts all discussions of the future of care work. For the reality is that the costs, however defined, have been until now borne disproportionately by those who do the caring, in effect subsidising those who do not. Tronto states the situation bluntly, arguing that:

> social and economic inequality are part of a 'vicious care circle' that exacerbates inequality, i.e. those with more resources have more access to better care and fewer care burdens, and the lack of adequate care resources and disproportionate care burdens disadvantages those with fewer resources from gaining more resources with which to narrow the gaps that make them unequal.
>
> (2004: 5)

This present situation is not just and, as we have implied already, it cannot continue. The future of care work, we believe, cannot avoid a redistribution of resources – from non-carers to carers and from men to women. The size of that redistribution is the main point at issue. It is a highly political point, being part of a politics of care that goes to the heart of what kind of societies our post-industrial states become.

Note

1   The latest Strategic Trends report from the Ministry of Defence Joint Doctrine and Concept Centre can be accessed at http://www.jdcc-strategictrends.org.

Appendix
Research summaries

Care Work in Europe

Care Work in Europe: Current Understandings and Future Directions took place between 2001 and 2005 and was funded by the European Union as part of its 5th Framework Programme. It had six partners in Denmark, Hungary, the Netherlands, Spain, Sweden and the UK. The UK partners were the coordinators. The overall objective was to contribute to the development of good quality employment in caring services that are responsive to the needs of rapidly changing societies and their citizens. The project had three stages: mapping and review of paid care work in services for young children, children and young people, disabled adults and older people; three case studies of policy, training and practice that each took place in three or four countries and concerned work with young children; work with older people and work with severely disabled adults. Also in the second stage was a study developing a cross-national video observation method called Sophos. The last stage was a dissemination phase and also involved documenting innovative practice in the six countries. Reports from all stages of the work are available on the project website www.ioe.ac.uk/tcru/carework.htm.

Childminding in the 1990s

Who Cares? Childminding in the 1990s (Mooney et al. 2001) was a study funded by the Joseph Rowntree Foundation under their Work and Family Life Programme, to look at childminding as an occupation and its role in the provision of childcare and took place between 1999 and 2000. The research involved secondary analysis of the Family Resource Survey; a postal survey of a nationally representative sample of 1,050 childminders drawn from eight English authorities; and case studies of 10 new, 10 established and 10 former childminders from two contrasting English authorities. Parents using the 20 new and established case study childminders were interviewed by telephone. A short extension to the initial study (the findings of which were included in the above publication) considered the reasons for the documented national fall in the number of childminders. This work involved secondary analysis of government statistics, a survey of Early Years Development and Childcare Partnerships and interviews with key officers from the National Childminding Association and ten local authorities showing a significant drop in the number of registered childminders.

The Fifty Plus study

The Pivot Generation: Informal Care and Work after Fifty (Mooney et al. 2002) was funded by the Joseph Rowntree Foundation and took place between 2000 and 2002. It looked at how decisions about employment are influenced by the desire or need to provide informal care for grandchildren or elderly relatives. Informal care was defined as regularly (at least once a month) looking after grandchildren while their parents worked or studied, or providing care/help for elderly or disabled relatives, neighbours or friends. The study had three stages: the first two were secondary analysis of the Labour Force Survey between 1979 and 1999 and looked at changes over time in employment patterns at household level and the implications of this for the availability of people in their fifties and sixties to provide care; and a postal survey completed by over 1,000 employees aged 50 or over and recent retirees, from one urban and one rural English local authority (representing a response rate of 38 per cent). The aim of the survey was to provide information on the extent to which older workers have caring responsibilities or will have in the future, who they care for and what they do. Of particular interest was the impact their caring responsibilities may have on their lives especially paid work. The third stage was in-depth interviews carried out with 22 carers and 10 non-carers to explore how informal care and other factors affected decisions about paid work. Interviewees were providing care to different people (elderly relatives, grandchildren, own children, spouse, friends and neighbours) and some had multiple care responsibilities whilst others undertook just one type of care.

The Foundling Hospital study

The Foundling Hospital Study (Oliver 2003; Oliver and Aggleton 2000) took place between 1997 and 1998 and was funded by the Nuffield Foundation. It was a pilot project based on the Thomas Coram Foundling Hospital, a charitable institution set up in the eighteenth century which aimed to provide care for the many illegitimate babies who, at that time, were abandoned and left to die on the streets of London. The Foundling Hospital evolved a phased system of care, linked to the age of the child, which remained largely unchanged until the 1940s. In 1997, twenty-five former pupils of the Foundling Hospital born between 1900 and 1955 were interviewed about their childhood memories. Of the 25 adults interviewed, 13 were women and 12 were men. Collectively, their childhoods spanned the three main locations of the Foundling Hospital, from London (until 1926), to Redhill (1926–34) and finally Berkhamsted (1934–53).

Four Generation study

Working and Caring over the Twentieth Century (Brannen et al. 2004) was funded by the Economic and Social Research Council and explored the process of change and continuity in employment and care across the life course of men and women in four-generation families and took place between 1999 and 2000. It focused specifically on the care they give and receive from family members and their employment practices over the life course phases of parenthood and considered both intra and intergenerational relations. Twelve case study families were chosen where the youngest adult generation had a young child. Interviews using biographical methods were undertaken with the three adult generations in each family, referred to in the study as the great grandparent, grandparent and parent generation. Altogether, 71 family members were interviewed and their life stories span much of the twentieth century and the social change that has occurred during this century.

Mapping the Social Care Workforce study

Mapping the Care Workforce: Supporting joined-up thinking; Secondary analysis of the Labour Force Survey for childcare and social care work (Simon et al. 2003) was conducted between 2001 and 2002 using data from the spring quarters of the Labour Force Survey for the years 1997, 1998 and 1999. The Labour Force Survey (LFS) is a large government survey of 60,000 households in the UK each quarter. The care workforce was defined using the Office for National Statistics' Standard Occupational Classification, and a number of characteristics about the care workforce were analysed, including gender, ethnicity, age, living and working arrangements and pay. Comparisons were conducted with education and nursing workers, as well as with occupations characterised by high levels of female workers, and with all women workers. The study was conducted for the Department of Health, and material from the Labour Force Survey is Crown Copyright, made available with permission by the Office for National Statistics through the UK Data Archive.

Men in the Nursery

Men in the Nursery: Gender and Caring Work (Cameron et al. 1999) took place between 1997 and 1999 and was funded by the Department of Health and the Department for Education and Skills. Its main objective was to better understand why the staffing of childcare services in England is so gendered. The study adopted a multi-method approach including a survey of further education college lecturers, secondary analysis of large-scale data sets, and an in-depth interview study of 21 male and female childcare workers in ten childcare centres.

The Mentoring study

National Evaluation of Youth Justice Board Round 8 Mentor Projects (St James-Roberts et al. 2004a), took place between 2001 and 2005 and was funded by the Youth Justice Board (YJB). At the end of 2001, 84 projects across England and Wales were funded by the YJB to set up mentor projects designed to reduce offending in young people. This study aimed to support the projects and to evaluate their effectiveness. By September 2003, the projects had recruited 2,393 mentors and 2,843 young people, and had set up 1,486 mentoring programmes. An interim report, submitted to the YJB at that stage is available by request from the authors. The final report, due in 2005, will identify the features of projects and young people that lead to successful outcomes.

The Private Fostering study

The *Private Fostering* study took place between 2002 and 2004 and was funded by the Department Health, following their publication of a booklet entitled *Private Fostering: A Cause for Concern* (Department of Health 2001b). Very little is known about private fostering. This project aimed to investigate the motivations and experiences of those involved in private fostering, including the foster carers, the parents and people who have been privately fostered. Foster carers were identified mostly through social workers: 29 were interviewed. Young adults who had been privately fostered as children were contacted through a number of means, including articles in newspapers: 12 were interviewed. Parents proved much more difficult to contact: only three agreed to be interviewed.

Social Pedagogy 1 and *Social Pedagogy 2*

Social Pedagogy and Looked After Children in Five European Countries, and the *Social Pedagogic Approach in Relation to the Quality of Life and Life Chances of Looked After Children in Denmark, France and Germany* (Petrie et al. forthcoming) are two studies that took place between 2000 and 2004, funded originally by the Department of Health, and subsequently the Department for Education and Skills. They aimed firstly to explore the pedagogic approach in relation to residential care in the five countries, and secondly to compare the experiences of staff and young people in residential care establishments in other countries with that in England. *Social Pedagogy 1* used a comparative case study approach; interviews were conducted with policy-makers, teachers and students of pedagogy, and practitioners who work with children in residential settings. Comparative analyses explored similarities and differences of approach using pedagogic principles and strategies. These analyses were then considered within the British context, to explore the ways in which a pedagogic approach might inform UK policies for looked after children. *Social Pedagogy* 2 used a mixed quantitative and qualitative survey design in 52 residential homes in England, Denmark and Germany. The survey combined closed and open-ended questions and assessed the organisation of and daily practice in residential care from the perspectives of heads of establishment (N = 52), residential care workers (N = 139) and young people (N = 302).

The Sponsored Day Care study

The *Sponsored Day Care* study (Statham et al. 2001) was funded by the Department of Health and took place between 1996 and 2000. It explored the social work practice of purchasing places in independent day care services (childminders, playgroups and day nurseries) to support families experiencing difficulties. The project investigated the extent to which local authorities in England were providing this service, how it was organised, and its effectiveness in supporting children in need from the perspective of parents, social workers and day care providers. A multi-method approach was adopted utilising both qualitative and quantitative methods, including a postal survey of all English social services departments, secondary analysis of government day care statistics, visits to 12 local authorities operating day care placement schemes, document and records analysis, face-to-face interviews with local authority staff, parents and childminders, and observation of meetings and of childminding placements.

References

Aldgate, J. and Bradley, M. (1999) *Supporting Families Through Short-term Fostering*, London: The Stationery Office.

Alexander, E. (2002) 'Childcare Students: Learning or Imitating?' *Forum*, 44: 24–6.

Andersen, B. (2000) *Doing the Dirty Work? The Global Politics of Domestic Labour*, London: Zed Books.

ARTD (2002) *Mentoring for Young Offenders: Final Report of the NSW Pilot Program*, Haberfield, NSW, Australia: Crime Prevention Division, Attorney General's Department & Department of Juvenile Justice, NSW Government.

Barreau, S. (2004) 'On Their Own', *Community Care*, 38–9.

Barrow, C. (1996) *Family in the Caribbean: Themes and Perspectives*, Oxford: J. Currey.

Barry, M. (2000) 'The Mentor/Monitor Debate in Criminal Justice: "What works" for Offenders?' *British Journal of Social Work*, 30: 575–95.

Bebbington, A. and Miles, J. (1990) 'The Supply of Foster Families for Children in Care', *British Journal of Social Work*, 20: 283–307.

Beck, U. (1998) *Democracy: What Enemies*, Cambridge: Polity Press.

Berridge, D. (1994) 'Foster and Residential Care Reassessed: A Research Perspective', *Children and Society*, 8, 2: 132–50.

Berridge, D., ed. (1997) *Foster Care: A Research Review*. London: The Stationery Office.

Berridge, D. and Brodie, I. (1997) *Children's Homes Revisited*, London: Jessica Kingsley.

Big Brothers Big Sisters Website.
http://www.bbbsa.org/site/pp.asp?c=iuJ3JgO2F&b=14600 (accessed 10 Nov 2004)

Boddy, J., Marjorie, S. and Simon, A. (2004) *Evaluation of Parentline Plus. Home Office Online Report 33/04*, London: Home Office.

Bostock, L. (2003) *Effectiveness of Childminding Registration and its Implications for Private Fostering*, London: SCIE.

Brannen, J. and Moss, P., eds (2003) *Rethinking Children's Care*, Buckinghamshire: Open University Press.

Brannen, J., Moss, P. and Mooney, A., eds (2004) *Working and Caring Over the Twentieth Century: Change and Continuity in Four Generation Families*, London: Palgrave Macmillan.

Brontë, C. (1953) *Jane Eyre*, Harmondsworth: Penguin Books Ltd.

Brookes, R., Regan, S. and Robinson, P. (2002) *A New Contract for Retirement*, London: Institute for Public Policy Research.

Brophy, J., Statham, J. and Moss, P. (1992) *Playgroups in Practice: Self Help and Public Policy*, London: HMSO.

Brown, B., Nolan, P. and Crawford, P. (2000) 'Men in Nursing: Ambivalence in Care, Gender and Masculinity', *International History of Nursing Journal*, 5: 4–13.

Burdett-Coutts, A. (1979) 'A Letter to the English Journal of Education, 1858', *Women in Public: 1850–1900 Documents of the Victorian Women's Movement*, London: George Allan and Unwin.

Cabinet Office Strategy Unit (2002) *Delivering for Children and Families: Interdepartmental Childcare Review*, London: Cabinet Office Strategy Unit.

Cameron, C. (1999) *Child Protection and Independent Day Care Services: Examining the Interface of Policy and Practice*, London: Institute of Education University of London.

Cameron, C. (2003) *A Historical Perspective on Changing Child Care Policy*, Buckingham: Open University Press.

Cameron, C. (2004) 'Social Pedagogy and Care: Danish and German Practice in Young People's Residential Care', *Journal of Social Work*, 4: 133–51.

Cameron, C., Moss, P. and Owen, C. (1999) *Men in the Nursery: Gender and Caring Work*, London: Paul Chapman Publishing.

Cameron, C., Owen, C. and Moss, P. (2001) *Entry, Retention and Loss: A Study of Childcare Students and Workers. DfES Research Report 275*, London: DfES.

Cameron, C. and Phillips, J. (2003a) *Case Study of Care Work in Residential and Home Care*. London: Thomas Coram Research Unit, Institute of Education, University of London.

Carers UK (2001) *It Could Be You: A Report on the Chances of Becoming a Carer*. London: Carers UK.

Carers UK (2002) *Without Us*. London: Carers UK.

Carew, R. (1979) 'The Place of Knowledge in Social Work Activity', *British Journal of Social Work*, 9: 349–64.

Chase, E., Simon, A. and Jackson, S., eds (forthcoming) *In Care and After: A Positive Perspective*. London: Routledge.

Christ, C. (1977) 'Victorian Masculinity and the Angel in the House', in M. Vicinus (ed.) *A Widening Sphere, Changing Roles of Victorian Women*, London: Methuen and Co Ltd.

Clarke, A., McQuail, S. and Moss, P. (2003) *Exploring the Field of Listening to and Consulting Young Children*. London: Department for Education and Skills.

Clough, R., Bullock, R., Ward, A., Colton, M., Pithouse, A., Roberts, S. and Ward, H. (2004) *Review of the Purpose and Future Shape of Fostering and Residential Care Services for Children in Wales*, Cardiff: National Assembly of Wales.

Clutterbuck, D. (2001) 'Twelve Habits of the Toxic Mentor', http://www.coaching-network.org.uk/ResourceCentre.htm (date accessed 16 June 2005).

Cohen, B., Moss, P., Petrie, P. and Wallace, J. (2004) *A New Deal for Children? Re-forming Education and Care in England, Scotland and Sweden*, Bristol: Polity Press.

Colley, H. (2003) *Mentoring for Social Inclusion: A Critical Approach to Nurturing Mentor Relationships*, London and New York: RoutledgeFalmer.

Colton, M. (1992) 'Carers of Children: A Comparative Study of the Practices of Residential and Foster Carers', *Children and Society*, 6: 25–37.

Commission for Social Care Inspection (2004) 'Childrens' Homes by Sector', personal communication.

Commission on the Future of the Voluntary Sector (1996) *Meeting the Challenge of Change*, London: National Council for Voluntary Organisations.

Community Care (2003) 'News Analysis of Battle Councils Face to Keep Foster Carers', *Community Care*, 8 May 2003.

Connell, J. P., Kubisch, A. C., Schorr, L. B. and Wiess, C. H. (1995) *New Approaches to Evaluating Community Initiatives: Concepts, Methods and Contexts*, Washington, DC: The Aspen Institute.

Connexions Service National Unit and the Youth Justice Board (2001) *Working Together: Connexions and Youth Justice Services*. Nottingham: DfES Publications, Nottingham NG15 0DJ.

Coomans, G. (2002) 'Labour Supply in a European Context: Demographic Determinants and Competence Issues', paper given at European Conference on Employment Issues on the Care of Children and Older People Living at Home, Sheffield Hallam University, 22 June.

Cordeaux, C., Hall, B, Owen, S and Miles, R (1999) *HERA2: Final Report Child Care Training in the United Kingdon*, Ipswich: Suffolk County Council Social Services.

Cost Quality and Outcomes Study Team (1995) *Cost, Quality and Child Outcomes in Child Care Centers: Public Report*, Denver, Colorado: University of Colorado-Denver.

Dahlberg, G. (2000) 'Everything is a Beginning and Everything is Dangerous: Some Reflections on the Reggio Emilia Experience', in H. Penn (ed.) *Early Childhood Services: Theory, Policy and Practice*, Buckingham: Open University Press.

Dahlberg, G., Moss, P. and Pence, A. (1999) *Beyond Quality in Early Childhood Education and Care: Postmodern Perspectives on the Problem with Quality*, London: Falmer Press.

Daly, M. and Lewis, J. (1999) 'Introduction: Conceptualising Social Care in the Context of Welfare State Restructuring', in J. Lewis (ed.) *Gender, Social Care and the State Restructuring in Europe*, Aldershot: Ashgate.

Davison, A. (1995) *Residential Care: The Provision of Quality Care in Residential and Educational Group Care Settings*, Aldershot: Arena.

Dench, G. and Ogg, J. (2002) *Grandparenting in Britain: A Baseline Study*, London: Institute of Community Studies.

Department for Education and Skills (2001a) *Children's Homes at 31 March 2000 England*, London: The Stationery Office.

Department for Education and Skills (2001b) 'Statistics of Education: Children's Day Care Facilities at 31 March 2001 England'.

Department for Education and Skills (2003a) *Every Child Matters. Cm 5860*, London: The Stationery Office.

Department for Education and Skills (2003b) *Statistics of Education: Children Looked After by Local Authorities Year Ending 31 March 2003 Volume 1: Commentary and National Tables*.

Department of Education and Employment (1998) *Meeting the Childcare Challenge*, London: The Stationery Office.

Department for Education and Skills (2004a) *Children Looked After by Local Authorities Year Ending 31 March 2003 England*, London: The Stationery Office.

Department for Education and Skills (2004b) *Five Year Strategy for Children and Learners*. London: Department for Education and Skills.

Department for Education and Skills (2005) 'Enhancement of Private Fostering Notification System: Consultation', Department for Education and Skills.

Department for Education and Skills, Department of Health and Home Office (2003) *Keeping Children Safe: The Government's Response to the Victoria Climbié Inquiry Report and Joint Chief Inspectors' Report Safeguarding Children. Cm 5861*, London: The Stationery Office.

Department of Health (1991a) *The Children Act 1989 Guidance and Regulations. Volume 8: Private Fostering and Miscellaneous*, London: HMSO.

Department of Health (1991b) *The Children Act Guidance and Regulations, Vol 2: Family Support, Day Care and Educational Provision for Young Children*, London: HMSO.

Department of Health (1998) *Modernising Social Services*, London: The Stationery Office.

Department of Health (1999) *National Strategy for Carers*, London: Department of Health.

Department of Health (2001a) *National Service Framework for Older People*, London: Department of Health.

Department of Health (2001b) *Private Fostering. A Cause for Concern*. London: Department of Health.

Department of Health (2002a) *Children's Homes, National Minimum Standards Children's Homes Regulations*. London: The Stationery Office.

Department of Health (2002b) *National Minimum Standards for Children's Homes*, London: Department of Health.

Department of Health (2003a) *Care Homes for Older People, National Minimum Standards*, London, The Stationery Office. London: Department of Health.

Department of Health (2003b) *Domicilary Care, National Minimum Standards, Regulations*.

Department of Health and Department for Education and Skills (2004) *National Service Framework for Children, Young People and Maternity Services*, London: Department of Health.

Dickens, C. (Undated (a)) *Nicholas Nickleby*, London: The Educational Book Company.

Dickens, C. (Undated (b)) *Martin Chuzzlewit*, London: The Educational Book Company.

Dickens, C. (Undated (c)) *Oliver Twist*, London: The Educational Book Company.

Dickens, C. (Undated (d)) *David Copperfield*, London: The Educational Book Company.

Dickens, C. (Undated (e)) *Bleak House*, London: The Educational Book Company.

Dickens, C. (Undated (f)) *Our Mutual Friend*, London: The Educational Book Company.

Dupree, E., Bertram, T. and Pascal, C. (2001) *Listening to Children's Perspectives on their Early Childhood Settings*. European conference on quality in early childhood education, Alkmaar Netherlands.

Eborall, C. (2003) *The State of the Social Care Workforce in England, Volume 1 of the First Annual Report of the TOPPS England Workforce Intelligence Unit*. Leeds: Topps England.

Eborall, C. and Garmeson, K. (2001) *Desk Research on Recruitment and Retention in Social Care and Social Work*, COI communications for the Department of Health.

Edmond, R. (2003) 'Putting the Care into Residential Care: The Role of Young People', *Journal of Social Work*, 3, 3: 321–37.

Edwards, L. and Hatch, B. (2003) *Passing Time: A Report About Young People and Communities*, London: Institute for Public Policy Research.

Eliot, G. (1984) *Daniel Deronda*, Oxford: Oxford University Press.

Eliot, G. (1996) *Silas Marner*, London: Penguin.

Elliott, S. (2003) 'The Influence of Size of a Residential Establishment on Practice', *Children webmag*.

European Network of Youth and Child Mentoring Organizations (2004) http://www.enymo.homestead.com/pageensiteplan.html (date accessed 16 June 2005).

Esping-Andersen, G. (1999) *Social Foundations of Postindustrial Economies*, Oxford: Oxford University Press.

Evandrou, M. (1995) 'Employment and Care, Paid and Unpaid Work: The Socio-Economic Position of Informal Carers in Britain', in J. Phillips (ed.) *Working Carers: International Perspectives on Working and Caring for Older People*, Aldershot: Avebury.

Evandrou, M. (2003) 'Combining Work and Family Life: The Pension Penalty of Caring', *Ageing and Society*, 23: 583–601.

Everiss, L. and Dalli, C. (2003) 'Family Day Care in New Zealand: Training, Quality and Professional Status', *Family Day Care; Internatonal Perspectives on Policy, Practice and Quality*, London: Jessica Kingsley.

Ewijk, H. van (2005) 'Characteristics of Care and Social Work', *European Journal of Social Work*, 7: 83–89.

Ewijk, H., van Hens, H., Lemmersen, G. and Moss, P. (2002a) *Mapping of Care Services and the Care Workforce: Summary of Consolidated Report*, London: Thomas Coram Research Unit.

Ewijk, H., van Lammersen, G. and Moss, P. (2002b) *Mapping of Care Services and the Care Workforce: Consolidated report*, London: Thomas Coram Research Unit, Institute of Education, University of London, http://www.ioe.ac.uk/tcro/carework (date accessed 16 June 2005).

Farrington, D. P. (1989) 'Self-reported and Official Offending from Adolescence to Adulthood', in M. W. Klein (ed.) *Cross National Research in Self-Reported Crime and Delinquency*, Dordecht: Kluwer.

Farrington, D. P. (1996) *Understanding and Preventing Youth Crime*, York: Joseph Rowntree Foundation.

Finch, J. (1989) *Family Obligations and Social Change*, Cambridge: Polity Press.

Fostering Network (2003) *Fostered Children Living on Less than Recommended Minimum*, http://www.thefostering.net/news/?article=3091501 (date accessed 16 June 2005).

Fostering Network (2005) *Minimum Allowances*, http://www.thefostering.net/campaigns/allowances/minimum.php (date accessed 17 June 2005).

Foucalt, M. (1988) *Politics, Philosophy, Culture: Interviews and Other Writings 1977–1984*, London: Routledge.

Francis, J. and Netten, A. (2003) *Home Care Workers: Careers, Commitments and Motivations*, Personal Social Services Research Unit, Discussion Paper 2053.

Frost, N., Johnson, L., Stein, M. and Wallis, L. (1996) *Negotiated Friendship: Home Start and the Delivery of Family Support*, Leicester: Home-Start UK.

Gardner, R. (2002) *Supporting Families: Child Protection in the Community*, Chichester: Wiley.

Gaskell, E. (1967) *Ruth*, London: J M Dent & Sons Ltd.

Ghate, D. and Ramella, M. (2002) *Positive Parenting: The National Evaluation of the Youth Justice Board's Parenting Programme*. Policy Research Bureau for the Youth Justice Board.

Godfrey, A. (2000) 'What Impact Does Training have on the Care Received by Older People in Residential Homes?' *Social Work Education*, 19: 55–65.

Goody, E. N. (1982) *Parenthood and Social Reproduction: Fostering and Occupational Roles in West Africa*, Cambridge: Cambridge University Press.

Goody, E. N. and Groothues, C. M. (1979) 'Stress in Marriage: West African Couples in London', in V. Saifullah Khan (ed.) *Minority Families in Britain*, London: Macmillan.

Gorham, D. (1982) *The Victorian Girl and the Feminine Ideal*, London: Croom Helm.

Graham, J. and Bowling, B. (1995) *Young People and Crime*. London: Home Office Research Study 145.

Green, H. (1988) *Informal Carers: A Study Carried out on behalf of the Department of Health and Social Security as part of the 1985 General Household Survey*, London: HMSO.

Greenfields, M. and Statham, J. (2004) *Support Foster Care: Developing a Short Break Service for Children in Need*, London: Institute of Education.

Greenwood, E. (1957) 'Social Work Research: A Decade of Reappraisal', *Social Service Review*, 31: 311–20.

Grossman, J. and Tierney, J. (1998) 'Does Mentoring Work? An Impact Study of the Big Brothers Big Sisters Program', *Evaluation Review*, 22: 403–26.

Grundy, E., Murphy, M. and Shelton, N. (1999) 'Looking Beyond the Household: Intergenerational Perspectives on Living Kin and Contact with Kin in Great Britain', *Population Trends*, 97: 19–27.

Gustavsson, A. (1996) *Tyst Kunskap – What is Tacit Knowledge?* Stockholm: Rapport fran CKVO – seminariet Pedagogiska Institutionen, Stockhoolm Universitet.

Halpern, D. (2003) *Social Capital and social software*, www.theworkfoundation.com/pdf/david_halpern.pdf (date accessed 16 June 2005).

Hämäläinen, J. (2003) 'The Concept of Social Pedagogy in the Field of Social Work', *Journal of Social Work*, 3: 69–80.

Hammerton, J. A. (Undated) *Life of Charles Dickens*, London: Chatto and Windus.

Henthorne, K. and Harkins, J. (2004) *Parents' Demand for and Access to Childcare in Scotland. Insight 13*, Edinburgh: Scottish Executive Education Department.

Heron, G. and Chakrabarti, M. (2002) 'Impact of Scottish Vocational Qualifications on Residential Child Care: Have they Fulfilled the Promise', *Social Work Education*, 21: 183–97.

Hevey, D. and Curtis, A. (1996) 'Training to Work in the Early Years', in G. Pugh (ed.) *Contemporary Issues in the Early Years: Working Collaboratively for Children*, London: Paul Chapman Publishing.

Hine, J. and Harrington, V. (2004) *Delivering On Track. Development and Practice Report*, London: Home Office.

Hochschild, A. (2000) 'Global Care Chains and Emotional Surplus Value', in W. Hutton and A. Giddens (eds) *On the Edge: Living with Global Capitalism*, London: Jonathan Cape.

Hollis, P. (1979) *Women in Public: 1850–1900, Documents of the Victorian Women's Movement*, London: George Allen and Unwin.

Holman, R. (1973) *Trading in Children: A Study of Private Fostering*, London: Routledge and Kegan Paul.

Holman, R. (2002) *The Unknown Fostering: A Study of Private Fostering*, Lyme Regis: Russell House.

Homer (800BC) *The Odyssey*. http://classics.mit.edu/Homer/odyssey.1.i.html (date accessed 16 June 2005).

Hutton, S. and Hirst, M. (1999) *Informal Care Giving in the Life Course: Caring Relationships Over Time*, York: Social Policy Research Unit University of York.

Improvement and Development Agency (1999) *Independent Sector Children's Residential Homes Survey 1998*. London: Employers' Organization.

Jensen, J. and Hansen, H. (2003a) *Danish National Report for Workpackage 7: Care Work in Europe*. Unpublished report, Aarhus, Jydskpædagogic Seminarium.

Johansson, S. (2002) *Den Sociala Omsorgens Akademisering. (Academization of Social Care Knowledge)*, Stockholm: Liber.

Johansson, S. and Moss, P. (2004) *Work with Elderly People: A Case Study of Sweden Spain and England with Additional Material from Hungary*, Thomas Coram Research Unit.

Jones, C. (1996) 'Anti-intellectualism and the Peculiarties of British Social Work Education', in N. Parton (ed.) *Social Theory, Social Change and Social Work*, London: Routledge.

Joseph, A. and Hallman, B. (1998) 'Over the Hill and Far Away: Distance as a Barrier to the Provision of Assistance to Elderly Relatives', *Social Science and Medicine*, 46: 631–9.

Joshi, H. (1995) 'The Labour Market and Unpaid Caring: Conflict and Compromise', in I. Allen and E. Perkins (eds) *The Future of Family Care for Older People*, London: HMSO.

Karllson, M. (2003) 'The Everyday Life of Children in Family Day Care as seen by their Carers', *Family Day Care: International Perspectives on Policy, Practice and Quality*, London: Jessica Kingsley Publishers.

Kendall, J. (2000) 'The Mainstreaming of the Third Sector into Public Policy in England in the late 1990s: Whys and Wherefores', *Policy and Politics*, 28: 541–62.

Kitwood, Y. (1998) 'Professional and Moral Development for Care Work: Some Observations on the Process', *Journal of Moral Education*, 27: 401–11.

Knapp, M., Koutsogeorgopoulou, V. and Smith, J. D. (1995) *Who Volunteers and Why? The Key Factors which Determine Volunteering*, London: Volunteer Centre UK.

Kodz, J., Kersley, B. and Bates, P. (1999) *The Fifties Revival*, Brighton: Institute for Employment Studies.

Korintus, M. (2003) 'Some Unique Features of the Emerging Family Day Care Provision in Hungary: Home Like?' *Family Day Care: International Perspectives on Policy, Practice and Quality*, London: Jessica Kingsley Publishers.

Korintus, M. and Moss, P. (2003) *Work with Young Children: A Case Study of Denmark, Hungary and Spain, Consolidated Report*. London: Thomas Coram Research Unit, Institute of Education, University of London, http.//www.ioe.ac.uk/tcro/carework (accessed 16 June 2005).

Kröger, T. (2001) *Comparative Research on Social Care: The State of the Art*. Brussels: European Commision.

La Valle, I., Arthur, S., Millward, C., Scott, J. and Clayden, M. (2002) *Happy Families? Atypical Work and its Influence on Family Life*, Bristol: Policy Press.

Laing and Buisson (2004) *Long Term Care*. http://www.laingbuisson.co.uk/longtermcare.htm (accessed 16 June 2005).

Laming, R. (2003) *The Victoria Climbié Inquiry*. CM 5730, London: HMSO.

Li, M. (2005) 'Towards Equal Voices: Childcare and Children in Chinese and Bangladeshi Households in Newcastle Upon Tyne', Newcastle Upon Tyne: University of Newcastle Upon Tyne.

Lingsom, S. (1997) 'The Substitution Issue: Care Policies and their Consequences for Family Care', *NOVA Norwegian Social Research*, Oslo.

Lipsey, M. (1995) 'What do We Learn from 400 Research Studies on the Effectiveness of Treatment with Juvenile Delinquents', in J. McGuire (ed.) *What Works: Reducing Reoffending*: Wiley.

Loeber, R. (1990) 'Development and Risk Factors of Juvenile Antisocial Behaviour and Delinquency', *Clinical Psychology Review*, 10: 1–41.

Lyon, D. (2004) 'The Interconnectedness of Care Work', paper given at a workshop, Transformations of Work: Gendered Labour and the Shifting Boundaries Between Unpaid and Paid Work, Robert Schuman Centre for Advanced Studies, European University Institute, Florence.

Macfarlane, A. (1993) *The Right to Make Choices*, Basingstoke: Macmillan.

Maher, J. and Green, H. (2002) *Carers 2000: Results from the Carers Module of the General Household Survey 2000*, London: The Stationery Office.

McGill, D. E. (1999) 'Mentoring as an Early Intervention Strategy: The Experience of Big Brothers Big Sisters of America', in R. Bayley (ed.) *Transforming Children's Lives: the Importance of Early Intervention*, London: Family Policy Studies Centre.

McGonigle, T. (2002) 'The Contribution of Volunteers to Work with Children in a Criminal Justice Organisation', *Child Care in Practice*, 8: 262–72.

McKay, S. and Middleton, S. (1998) *Characteristics of Older Workers: Secondary Analysis of the Family and Working Lives*, London: DfEE.

Milham, S., Bullock, R. and Hose, K. (1980) *Learning to Care: The Training of Staff for Residential Social Work with Young People*, Farnborough: Gower.

Miltoun, F. (1904) *Dicken's London*, London: Eveleigh Nash.

Ministry of Defence (2005) *JDCC Strategic Trends*. London: Ministry of Defence.

Ministry of Health (1945) 'Circular', 221/45.

Ministry of Health (1968) 'Circular', 37/68.

Mooney, A. and Blackburn, T. (2003) *Children's Views on Childcare Quality*, London: Department for Education and Skills.

Mooney, A., Knight, A., Moss, P. and Owen, C. (2001) *Who Cares? Childminding in the 1990s*, London: Family Policy Studies Centre, Joseph Rowntree Foundation.

Mooney, A., Statham, J. and Simon, A. (2002) *The Pivot Generation: Informal Care and Work after 50*, Bristol: Policy Press.

Morris, J. (1993) *Community Care or Independent Living?* York: Joseph Rowntree Foundation.

Mortimore, P., ed. (1999) *Understanding Pedagogy and it's Impact on Learning*, London: Chapman.

Moss, P. (2003) 'Conclusion: Whither Family Day Care?' *Family Day Care: International Perspectives on Policy Practice and Quality*, London: Jessica Kingsley Publishers.

Moss, P. and Cameron, C. (2002) *Care Work and the Care Workforce: Report on Stage One and the State of the Art Review*, http://www.ioe.ac.uk/tcro/carework/reports (date accessed 16 June 2005).

Moss, P., Dillon, J. and Statham, J. (2000) 'The "Child in Need" and "the Rich Child": Discourses Constructions and Practice', *Critical Social Policy*, 20: 233–54.

Moss, P. and Petrie, P. (2002) *From Children's Service's to Children's Spaces*, London: Routledge Falmer.

Moyles, J. (2001) 'Passion, Paradox and Professionalism in Early Years Education', *Early Years*, 21: 81–95.

Mroz, M. and Hall, E. (2003) 'Not Yet Identified: The Knowledge, Skills and Training Needs of Early Years Professionals in Relation to Children's Speech and Language Development', *Early Years*, 23: 118–30.

Munton, T. and Zurawan, A. (2004) *Active Communities: Headline Findings from the 2003 Home Office Citizenship Survey*, London: Home Office.

National Archives Research Guides (2004a) *Civilian Nurses and Nursing Services*, www.catalogue.nationalarchives.gov.uk/rdleaflet.asp?sleafletID=121 (date accessed 16 June 2005).

National Archives Research Guides (2004b) *Royal Navy: Nurses and Nursing Services* www.catalogue.nationalarchives.gov.uk/rdleaflet.asp?sleafletID=51 (date accessed 16 June 2005).

Nelson, M. (1994) 'Family Day Care Providers: Dilemmas of Daily Practice', *Mothering: Ideology, Experience, Agency*, New York: Routledge.

New Zealand Ministry of Education (2002) 'Pathways for the Future: A Strategic Plan for Early Childhood Education', http://www.minedu.govt.nz (date accessed 16 June 2005).

Neysmith, S. M. and Aronson, J. (1996) 'Home Care Workers Discuss their Skills: The Skills required to "Use your Common Sense" ', *Journal of Aging Studies*, 10: 1–14.

O'Donnell, C. R., Lydgate, T. and Fo, W. S. O. (1979) 'The Buddy System: Review and Follow-up', *Child Behavior Therapy*, 1: 161–9.

Office for National Statistics (1999) *LFS User Guide*, London: ONS.

Office for National Statistics (2000) *Standard Occupational Classification 2000*, London: The Stationery Office.

Office for National Statistics (2003a) *Census 2001 National Report for England and Wales*, London: The Stationery Office.

Office for National Statistics (2003b) *Census 2001: Carers*, http://www.statistics.gov.uk/cci/nugget.asp?id=347 (date accessed 16 June 2005).

Office for National Statistics (2003c) *Social Trends: 2003 edition*, London: The Stationery Office.

Office for National Statistics (2004) *Consultation Paper: Proposals for a Continuous Population Survey*. London: National Statistics.

Office for Standards in Education (2001a) *Full Day Care: Guidance to the National Standards*, http://www.ofsted.gov.uk/publications/index.cfm?fuseaction.pubs.   summary@id=2427 (accessed 16 June 2005).

Office for Standards in Education (2001b) *Childminding: Guidance to the National Standards*, http://www.ofsted.gov.uk/publications/index.cfm?fuseaction=pubs.   summary@id=2435 (accessed 16 June 2005).

Oliver, C. (2003) 'The Care of the Illegitimate Child: The Coram Experience 1900–1945', *Rethinking Children's Care*, Buckingham: Open University Press.

Oliver, C. and Aggleton, P. (2000) *Coram's Children: Growing up in the Care of the Foundling Hospital 1900–1955*, London: Coram Family.

Organisation for Economic Co-operation and Development (2001) *Starting Strong*, Paris: OECD.

Owen, C. (1999) 'Government Household Surveys', in D. Dorling and S. Simpson (eds) *Statistics in Society*, London: Arnold.

Owen, S. (2003) 'The Development of Childminding Networks in Britain: Sharing the Caring', *Family Day Care: International Perspectives on Policy, Practice and Quality*, London: Jessica Kingsley Publishers.

Packman, J. and Hall, C. (1998) *From Care to Accommodation*, London: The Stationery Office.

Parker, R. (2003) The York Day: Size Matters. *Children Webmag*, http://www.childrenUK.co.uk/chjan2003/webmag.hfm (date accessed 28 June 2005).

Patmore, C. (1998) *The Angel in the House*, London: Haggerston Press with Boston College.

Peace, S. (1998) 'Caring in Place', in S. Peace (ed.) *Care Matters: Concepts, Practice and Research in Health and Social Care*, London: Sage.

Peterson, J. M. (1972) 'The Victorian Governess', in M. Vincinus (ed.) *Suffer and be Still: Women in the Victorian Age*, London: Methuen and Co Ltd.

Petrie, P. (1994) *Play and Care*, London: HMSO.

Petrie, P. (2003) 'Social Pedagogy: An Historical Account of Care and Education as Social Control', in J. Brannen and P. Moss (eds) *Rethinking Children's Care*, Buckingham: Open University Press.

Petrie, P., Boddy, J., Cameron, C. and Wigfall, V. (forthcoming) *Working with Children in Care: European Perspectives*, Maidenhead: Open University Press.

Philip, K. (2000) 'Mentoring: Pitfalls and Potential for Young People?', *Source Youth and Policy*, 67 Summer: 1–15.

Philip, K., King, C. and Shucksmith, J. (2004) *Sharing a Laugh? A Qualitative Study of Mentoring Interventions with Young People*, York: Joseph Rowntree Foundation.

Phillips, J. (1999) 'Developing a Caregivers' Strategy in Britain', in V. M. Lechner and M. B. Neal (eds) *Work and Caring for the Elderly: International Perspectives*, London: Brunner/Mazel.

Phillips, J., Bernard, M. and Chittendon, M. (2002) *Juggling Work and Care: The Experiences of Working Carers and Older Adults*, Bristol: Policy Press.

Philpot, T. (2001) *A Very Private Practice: An Investigation into Private Fostering*, London: BAAF.

Pickard, L. (2002) 'The Decline of Intensive Intergenerational Care of Older People in Great Britain 1985–1995', *Population Trends*, 110: 31–41.

Pinchbeck, I. and Hewitt, M. (1973) *Children in English Society*, London: Routledge and Kegan Paul.

Popple, K. and Redmond, M. (2000) 'Community Development and the Voluntary Sector in the New Millenium: The Implications of the Third Way in the UK', *Community Development Journal*, 35.

Qualifications and Curriculum Authority (2004) *National Occupational Standards*. http://www.qca.org.uk/adultlearning/workforce/2677.html (date accessed 16 June 2005).

Quality and Curriculum Authority (1999) *Early Years Education, Childcare and Playwork: A Framework of Nationally Accredited Qualifications*. London: QCA.

Reynolds, T. (2001) 'Black Mothering, Paid Work and Identity', *Ethnic and Racial Studies*, 24: 1046–64.

Rhodes, J., Bogat, G. A., Roffman, J., Edelman, P. and Galasso, L. (2002) 'Youth Mentoring in Perspective: Introduction to the Special Issue', *American Journal of Community Psychology*, 30: 149–55.

Rickards, L. (2004) *Living in Britain: No 31: Results from the 2002 General Household Survey*, London: The Stationery Office.

Rinaldi, C. (2005) *In Dialogue with Reggion Emilia*, London: Falmer Routledge.

Roberts, H., Liabo, K., Lucas, P., Dubois, D. I. and Sheldon, T. A. (2004) 'Mentoring to Address Anto-Social Behaviour in Childhood', *British Medical Journal*, 328: 512–14.

Roche, D. and Rankin, J. (2004) *Who Cares? Building the Social Care Workforce*, London: Institute for Public Policy and Research.

Sallnas, M., Vinnerljung, B. and Westermark, P. (2004) 'Breakdown of Teenage Placements in Swedish Residential and Foster Care', *Child and Family Social Work*, pp. 141–52.

Sargeant, A. (2000) 'An Exploratory Study of the Effects of Progression towards National Vocational Qualifications on the Occupational Knowledge and Care Practice of Social Care Workers', *Social Work Education*, 19: 639–61.

Sellick, C. and Connolly, J. (2001) *National Survey of Independent Fostering Agencies*, Norwich: University of East Anglia.

Shiner, M., Young, T., Newburn, T. and Groben, S. (2004) *Mentoring Disaffected Young People: An Evaluation of Mentoring Plus*, York: LSE and Joseph Rowntree Foundation.

Simon, A. and Owen, C. (2005) *Using the Labour Force Survey to Map the Care Workforce, Labour Market Trends, 113: 201–208*.

Simon, A., Owen, C., Moss, P. and Cameron, C. (2003) *Mapping the Care Workforce: Supporting Joined-up Thinking*, London: Institute of Education.

Sinclair, I. and Gibbs, I. (1998) *Children's Homes: A Study in Diversity*, Chichester: Wiley.

Sinclair, I., Gibbs, I. and Wilson, K. (2000) *Supporting Foster Placements: Reports One and Two*, York: Social Work Research and Development Unit.

Sinclair, I., Wilson, K. and Gibbs, I. (2004) *Foster Placements: Why they Succeed and Why they Fail*, London: Jessica Kingsley Publishers.

Sinclair, I., Gibbs, I. and Hicks, L. (2000) *The Management and Effectiveness of the Home Care Service*, York: Social Work Research and Development Group, The University of York.

Singer, E. (1992) *Child Care: The Psychology of Development*, London: Routledge.

Sipilä, J. and Kröger, T. (2004) 'European Families Stretched Between the Demands of Work and Care', *Social Policy and Administration*, 38: 557–64.

Skinner, C. (2003) *Running Around in Circles: Co-ordinating Childcare, Education and Work*, Bristol: The Policy Press.

Smith, M. (2003) 'Towards a Professional Identity and Knowledge Base: Is Residential Child Care still Social Work?' *Journal of Social Work*, 3: 235–52.

Smith, M., McKay, E. and Chakrabarti, M. (2004) What Works for Us – Boys' Views of their Experiences in a Former List D School, *British Journal of Special Education*. 31: 89–93.

Social Care Institute of Excellence (2004) *A New Vision for Adult Social Care: Responses to a Survey Conducted by the Social Care Institute for Excellence*, London: SCRE.

Social Services Inspectorate (1994) *Signposts: Findings From a National Inspection of Private Fostering*, London: Social Services Inspectorate.

Speiss, C. and Schneider, A. (2003) 'Interactions Between Care-giving and Paid Work Hours Among European Midlife Women 1994–1996', *Ageing and Society*, 23: 41–68.

Spencer, N. (2003) 'Parenting Programmes', *Archives of Disease in Childhood*, 88: 99–100.

St James-Roberts, I., Greenlaw, G. and Simon, A. (2004a) *National Evaluation of Youth Justice Board Round 8 Mentor Projects*, unpublished, London: Youth Justice Board.

St James-Roberts, I., Greenlaw, G., Simon, A. and Hurry, J. (2004b) *National Evaluation Of Youth Justice Board Round 8 Mentor Projects: Interim Report*, London: Thomas Coram Research Unit, London: Institute of Education.

St James-Roberts, I. and Singh, C. S. (2001) *Mentors for primary school children with behaviour problems: an evaluation of the CHANCE project: Findings*, Home Office Research Findings, Vol. 157, pages 1–4, http://www.homeoffice.gov.uk/rds/pdfs/r157.pdf (accessed 16 June 2005).

Statham, J. (2003) 'Provider and Parent Perspectives on Family Day Care for "Children in Need": A Third Party In-between', *Family Day Care: International perspectives on Policy, Practice and Quality*, London: Jessica Kingsley Publishers.

Statham, J., Dillon, J. and Moss, P. (2001) *Placed and Paid For: Supporting Families Through Sponsored Daycare*, London: The Stationery Office.

Statham, J. and Mooney, A. (2003) *Around the Clock: Childcare Services at Atypical Times*, Bristol: Policy Press.

SureStart (2004) *Childcare: Extending Protection and Broadening Support*, London: SureStart.

SureStart (2004) *Childcare and Early Years Workforce Surveys 2002/3: Day Nurseries and other Full-day Care Provision*, London: SureStart.

Sylva, K., Melhuish, E., Sammons, P., Siraj-Blatchford, I., Taggart, B. and Elliot, K. (2003) *The Effective Provision of Pre-School Education (EPPE) Project: Findings from the Preschool Period Summary of Findings*. London: Institute of Education.

Tarling, R., Burrows, J. and Clarke, A. (2001) *Dalston Youth Project Part II (11- to 14-year-olds): An Evaluation*. London: Home Office Research, Development and Statistics Directorate.

Tarling, R., Davison, T. and Clarke, A. (2004) *A Summary of the National Evaluation of the Youth Justice Board's Mentoring Projects*, London: Youth Justice Board.

Taylor, R. (2004) 'Extending Conceptual Boundaries: Work, Voluntary Work and Employment', *Work, Employment and Society*, 18: 29–49.

Thackeray, W. M. (Undated) *Vanity Fair*, London: Hodder and Stoughton.

Tizard, B., Moss, P. and Perry, J. (1976) *All Our Children*, London: Temple Smith.

Triseliotis, J., Borland, M. and Hill, M. (2000) *Delivering Foster Care*, London: British Agencies for Adoption and Fostering.

Trollope, A. (1925) *The Warden*, London: Robert Hayes Ltd.

Tronto, J. (1993) *Moral Boundaries: A Political Argument for the Ethics of Care*, London: Routledge.

Tronto, J. (2004) *Vicious Circles of Privatised Care. Rethinking Care Relations, Family Lives and Policies*, University of Leeds.

Uglow, J. (1993) *Elizabeth Garkell. A Habit of Stories*, London: Faber and Faber.

Ungerson, C. (1997) 'Social Politics and the Commodification of Care', *Social Politics*, 4: 362–81.

Utting, W. B. (1997) *People Like Us: The Report of the Review of the Safeguards for Children Living Away From Home*, London: The Stationery Office.

Vevers, S. (2003) 'Home Delivery', *Nursery World*. 8 May: 10–1.

Volunteer Tutors Organisation (2000) *A Good Pal To Me: Young People's Views of the Befriending (Mentoring) Scheme Delivered by Edinburgh Volunteer Tutors Organisation*, Edinburgh: Volunteer Tutors Organisation.

Wærness, K. (1980) 'Omsorgen som lonearbete – en begreppsdiskussion', *Kvinnovetenskaplig tidskrift*, 3: 6–17.

Wærness, K. (1982) *Women's Perspectives in Social Policy*, Oslo, Bergen and Tromso: Universitetsforlaget.

Wærness, K. (1984) 'The Rationality of Caring', *Economic and Industrial Democracy*, 5: 185–211.

Wærness, K. (1995) 'Den Hjemmebaserte Omsorgen i den Skandinaviske Velferdsstat. En offentlig tjeneste i Spenningsfeltet Mellom ulike Kulturere', in S. Johansson (ed.) *Sjukhus och hem som Arbetsplats. Omsorgsyrken I Norge, Sverige och Finland*, Stockholm and Oslo: Bonniers and Universitetsforlaget.

Wagner, G. (1979) *Barnardo*, London: Weidenfield and Nicolson.

Watson, E. and Mears, J. (1999) *Women, Work and Care of the Elderly*, Aldershot: Ashgate Publishing.

Wheelock, J. and Jones, K. (2002) ' "Grandparents are the Next Best Thing": Informal Childcare for Working Parents in Urban Britain', *Journal of Social Policy*, 31: 441–63.

Whitebook, M., Howes, C. and Phillips, D. (1989) *Who Cares? Child Care Teachers and the Quality of Care in America: Final Report of the National Child Care Staffing Fund*, Oakland California: Child Care Employee Report.

Williams, F. (2001) 'In and Beyond New Labour: Towards a New Political Ethics of Care', *Critical Social Policy*, 21: 467–93.

Williams, F. (2004) *Rethinking Families*, London: Calouste Gulbenkian Foundation.

Woodland, S., Miller, M. and Tipping, S. (2002) *Repeat Study of Parents' Demand for Childcare*. London: DfES.

Woolf, V. (1970) 'Professions for Women' in *Death of the Moth and other Essays*, New York: Harcourt Brace Jovanovich.

Yeandle, S., Gore, T. and Herrington, A. (1999) *Employment, Family and Community Activities: A New Balance for Women and Men*, Dublin: European Foundation for Living and Working Conditions.

Youth Justice Board (2004) 'Double Act', *Youth Justice Board News*: 12.

Zeira, A. and Rosen, A. (2000) 'Unraveling "Tacit Knowledge": What Social Workers do and Why they do it', *Social Service Review*, 103–23.

Ziehe, T. (1998) *Cultural Analysis: Youngsters, Education and Modernity*, Stockholm: Norsteds Forlag.

Index